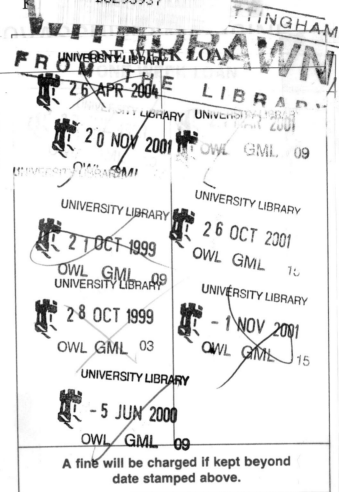

The KEY TOPICS Series

Advisors:

T.M. Craft *Department of Anaesthesia and Intensive Care, Royal United Hospital, Bath, UK*
C.S. Garrard *Intensive Therapy Unit, John Radcliffe Hospital, Oxford, UK*
P.M. Upton *Department of Anaesthetics, Treliske Hospital, Truro, UK*

Anaesthesia, Second Edition

Obstetrics and Gynaecology, Second Edition

Accident and Emergency Medicine

Paediatrics

Orthopaedic Surgery

Otolaryngology and Head and Neck Surgery

Ophthalmology

Psychiatry

General Surgery

Renal Medicine

Trauma

Chronic Pain

Oral and Maxillofacial Surgery

Oncology

Cardiovascular Medicine

Forthcoming titles include:
Paediatrics, Second Edition

Neonatology

Critical Care

Orthopaedic Trauma Surgery

Respiratory Medicine

Thoracic Surgery

KEY TOPICS IN
CARDIOVASCULAR MEDICINE

GREGORY Y.H. LIP
MD, MRCP, FACC, FESC
Consultant Cardiologist and Senior Lecturer in Medicine, University Department of Medicine and Department of Cardiology, City Hospital, Birmingham, UK

SHYAM P. SINGH
MD, FRCP
Consultant Cardiologist, Honorary Senior Clinical Lecturer in Cardiovascular Medicine and Examiner MRCP (UK) and PLAB Examinations, Department of Cardiology, City Hospital, Birmingham, UK

ROBERT D.S. WATSON
BSc, MD, FRCP
Consultant Cardiologist and Honorary Senior Clinical Lecturer in Cardiovascular Medicine, Department of Cardiology, City Hospital, Birmingham, UK

βIOS
SCIENTIFIC
PUBLISHERS
Oxford • Washington DC

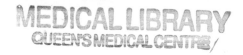
© BIOS Scientific Publishers Limited, 1998

First published 1998

A CIP catalogue record for this book is available from the British Library.

ISBN 1 85996 101 0   1 00161341 X

BIOS Scientific Publishers Ltd
9 Newtec Place, Magdalen Road, Oxford OX4 1RE, UK
Tel. +44 (0)1865 726286. Fax. +44 (0)1865 246823
World Wide Web home page: http://www.bios.co.uk/

DISTRIBUTORS

Australia and New Zealand
    Blackwell Science Asia
    54 University Street
    Carlton, South Victoria 3053

India
    Viva Books Private Limited
    4325/3 Ansari Road, Daryaganj
    New Delhi 110002

Singapore and South East Asia
    Toppan Company (S) PTE Ltd
    38 Liu Fang Road, Jurong
    Singapore 2262

USA and Canada
    BIOS Scientific Publishers
    PO Box 605, Herndon
    VA 20172-0605

Important Note from the Publisher
The information contained within this book was obtained by BIOS Scientific Publishers Ltd from sources believed by us to be reliable. However, while every effort has been made to ensure its accuracy, no responsibility for loss or injury whatsoever occasioned to any person acting or refraining from action as a result of information contained herein can be accepted by the authors or publishers.

The reader should remember that medicine is a constantly evolving science and while the authors and publishers have ensured that all dosages, applications and practices are based on current indications, there may be specific practices which differ between communities. You should always follow the guidelines laid down by the manufacturers of specific products and the relevant authorities in the country in which you are practising.

Production Editor: Andrea Bosher.
Typeset by Chandos Electronic Publishing, Stanton Harcourt, UK.
Printed by Redwood Books, Trowbridge, UK.

CONTENTS

[a]Contributed by S. Silverman, Consultant Vascular Surgeon, City Hospital, Dudley Road, Birmingham.

[b]Contributed by I. Goldsmith, Research Fellow in Cardiothoracic Surgery, Walesgrave Hospital, Coventry.

[c]Contributed by R. Patel, Consultant Cardiothoracic Surgeon, Walsgrave Hospital, Coventry.

[d]Contributed by I.F. Islim, Research Fellow in Cardiology, City Hospital, Dudley Road, Birmingham.

[e]Contributed by C. Gibbs, Research Fellow in Cardiology, City Hospital, Dudley Road, Birmingham.

[f]Contributed by V. Rathore, Research Fellow in Cardiology, City Hospital, Dudley Road, Birmingham.

[g]Contributed by P. Clarkson, Registrar in Cardiology, City Hospital, Dudley Road, Birmingham.

[h]Contributed by A. Notgi, Consultant in Nuclear Medicine, City Hospital, Dudley Road, Birmingham.

[i]Contributed by J. Gupta, Research Fellow in Cardiology, City Hospital, Dudley Road, Birmingham.

[j]Contributed by J. de Giovanni, Consultant Paediatric Cardiologist, Birmingham Children's Hospital, Ladywood, Birmingham.

[k]Contributed by D.G. Beevers, Professor of Medicine, City Hospital, Dudley Road, Birmingham.

ABBREVIATIONS

ABPI	ankle brachial pressure index
ACE	angiotensin converting enzyme
ADP	adenosine diphosphate
ANF	atrial naturetic factor
ASD	atrial septal defect
AV	atrioventricular
AVNRT	atrioventricular nodal re-entry tachycardias
AVRT	atrioventricular re-entrant tachycardia
CABG	coronary artery bypass graft
CCF	congestive cardiac failure
CHB	complete heart block
CT/MRI	computed tomography/magnetic resonance imaging
CXR	chest X-ray
DCM	dilated cardiomyopathy
DVT	deep vein thrombosis
ECG	electrocardiogram
EMF	endomyocardial fibrosis
ESR	erythrocyte sedimentation rate
HCM	hypertrophic cardiomyopathy
HDL	high density lipoproteins
IABP	intra-aortic balloon counterpulsion
IAT	intra-arterial thrombolysis
IDL	intermediate density lipoproteins
IE	infective endocarditis
INR	International Normalized Ratio
JVP	jugular venous pressure
LDL	low density lipoproteins
LVESD	left ventricular end-systolic dimension
LVH	left ventricular hypertrophy
MI	myocardial infarction
PE	pulmonary embolism
PSVT	paroxysmal supraventricular tachycardia
PTA	percutaneous transluminal angioplasty
PTCA	percutaneous transluminal coronary angioplasty
PVD	peripheral vascular disease
rTPA	recombinant tissue plasminogen activator
tPA	tissue plasminogen activator
VLDL	very low density lipoproteins
VSD	ventricular septal defect

PREFACE

This book is aimed at physicians in training, particularly those who are studying for their final examinations and higher professional examinations, such as the MRCP. This text should be used as an adjunct to the larger reference books. Topics have been selected to provide a broad base of knowledge in cardiovascular disease, with particular emphasis on important topics, difficult concepts, management problems and examination orientation. There is a standard format to each topic, with discussion on pathogenesis, identification and management.

Despite the many valued contributions from our colleagues, throughout the book we have attempted to achieve a constant style and to emphasise certain principles. We are grateful to our colleagues who have given helpful comments and ideas during the gestation of this text. We have taken care to try and exclude any factual errors and to include important recent advances in the key topics covered. Nevertheless, cardiovascular medicine is rapidly progressing and key references have been included to provide the reader with an insight into important recent literature. We sincerely hope that the reader finds the book a useful and valuable resource of knowledge of the key topics in cardiovascular medicine, not simply for approaching examinations but to apply many of the principles in their clinical practice.

G.Y.H. Lip
S.P. Singh
R.D.S. Watson

To Peck Lin, Indra and Ruth

SYMPTOMS AND SIGNS IN CARDIAC DISEASE

Symptoms in cardiac disease

Common symptoms
- Breathlessness (dyspnoea)
- Chest pain
- Palpitations
- Ankle swelling (oedema)

Less common symptoms
- Fainting (syncope)
- Cyanosis

Breathlessness

Sudden onset of breathlessness can be due to left ventricular failure. Elevated pulmonary venous pressure (pulmonary wedge, indirect left atrial/left ventricular end-diastolic pressure) results in escape of fluid in lung tissue which causes stiffness and subsequent increased effort of breathing. In this situation, lying flat may cause more discomfort in breathing and is called orthopnoea (due to increased venous return from the lower extremities, hence increasing the preload on the heart). Paroxysmal nocturnal dyspnoea is a symptom of left-sided cardiac failure. Breathlessness can also be a common symptom in pulmonary disease, severe anaemia and lack of cardiovascular fitness in sedentary lifestyle.

Chest pain

Cardiac ischaemia or anginal type pain occurs due to reduced myocardial oxygen supply or increased myocardial metabolic demands, consequent upon an increased heart rate provoked by physical exertion, acute stress or exposure to extremes of temperature, and is relieved by rest.

The common causes of non-cardiac chest pain are musculoskeletal aches, pleuritic pain or oesophageal reflux.

Palpitations

Awareness of heart beat is defined as palpitation. This may be functional, for example, in cases of insomnia or anxiety. Sudden, and often unprovoked, fast beating of the heart, lasting from a few minutes to hours, with abrupt relief, is due to paroxysmal tachyarrhythmias or atrial fibrillation. Brief sensation of missing heart beat followed by thumping sensation over the precordium, with sometimes pulsation in the neck, is due to extrasystoles.

Oedema

A common cause of oedema of the feet is venous insufficiency and it usually disappears in the morning. Oedema due to congestive cardiac failure is always accompanied by raised jugular venous pressure (JVP) and is a sign of right heart failure.

Syncope

Syncope usually occurs due to a vasovagal attack, e.g. prolonged standing or fright, arrhythmia, hypotension, vertebrobasilar ischaemia, or may be drug-induced, for example, with morphine. Syncope, due to severe aortic stenosis or hypertrophic obstructive cardiomyopathy, is usually provoked by physical effort. Complete heart block can also cause loss of consciousness, due to Stokes–Adams attack.

Vaso-vagal syncope is due to severe venodilation accompanied by bradycardia, resulting in low cardiac output and blood pressure. Postural hypotension may be a cause of syncope, and is often due to antihypertensive drugs. Micturition syncope is due to increased vagal tone. Severe prolonged coughing can similarly cause loss of consciousness (cough syncope). The increased intrathoracic pressure from coughing causes a Valsalva manoeuvre-type effect on cardiovascular haemodynamics, the venous return is reduced and there is a fall in cardiac output and blood pressure; after release of intrathoracic pressure, there is an increase in blood pressure. This physiological response is lacking in patients with cardiac failure and autonomic neuropathy, often seen in diabetics.

Cyanosis

Cyanosis is defined as the increased presence of deoxygenated haemoglobin at a concentration of >4g/dl, (O_2 saturation < 86%) resulting in the characteristic blue–purple appearance. Cyanosis may be central or peripheral.

Central cyanosis is due to reduced oxygenation of the blood and is noticed on the mucous membranes, including the lips, tongue and fingers; and is due to severe pulmonary disease or congenital cardiac disease with right to left shunt, e.g. Fallot's tetralogy.

Peripheral cyanosis is due to hypoperfusion and is noticed only in fingers or toes and can be due to cold extremities (acrocyanosis) or very low cardiac output state. Peripheral cyanosis can occur in isolation, but central cyanosis invariably leads to peripheral cyanosis.

The physical examination in cardiac patients

This should include inspection of hands to observe colour, evidence of clubbing or abnormality\ies in nails and fingers. Clubbing is seen in longstanding infective endocarditis and congenital cyanotic heart disease, but is also seen in thyrotoxicosis (thyroid acropachy), chronic liver disease, bronchial carcinoma, chronic lung infection (bronchiectasis, empyema, lung abscess) and malabsorption syndromes (including inflammatory bowel disease). Idiopathic clubbing is often familial and more pronounced.

Examination of hands may reveal splinter haemorrhages in nails, due to infective endocarditis or trauma. Osler's nodes are painful spots on fingers and similar lesions on palms are called Janeway spots. Red palms (palmar erythema) are seen in liver disease. Xanthomas are felt along tendons, and may be accompanied by corneal arcus (arcus senilis) which is seen in hyperlipidaemic states. Arachnodactyly is a manifestation of Marfan's syndrome.

Important physical signs. JVP is bilaterally raised in congestive cardiac failure or obstruction of superior vena cava, in the latter the venous pulse is not seen. JVP falls in inspiration and is more clearly seen during expiration. The reverse is seen in pericardial effusion/constriction and is called Kussmaul's sign. The wave form in JVP is similar to that in atrial tracing but only 'a' and 'v' waves are easily observed. Prominent 'a' waves occur in complete heart block and nodal and ventricular ectopics, when the atrium contracts during closed tricuspid valve (cannon waves). In tricuspid/severe pulmonary stenosis and pulmonary hypertension, large 'a' waves are easily observed. By contrast, 'a' waves are absent in atrial fibrillation. 'v' waves occur during atrial filling and are prominent in tricuspid regurgitation. Arterial carotid pulsation in the neck is often confused with venous pulsation, the latter, however, disappears on gentle pressure at the base of the neck. The hepatojugular reflex is not diagnostic of elevated JVP but helps to recognise the position of venous pulse.

Carotid pulsation can be seen in normal individuals but is accentuated in coarctation of aorta and when the arterial pulse pressure is high (high output state), for example, in aortic incompetence (Corrigan's pulse). A kinked carotid artery, which may be mistaken for aneurysm, occurs at the base of the neck, and mostly in females due to atheroma or hypertension.

The pulse. It is important to feel not only the radial but also the peripheral pulses. The essential features are:

- Rate.
- Rhythm.
- Character.
- Volume of pulse.

Irregular pulse:

- Sinus arrhythmia – in children and young adults – disappears with exercise.
- Atrial fibrillation – more apparent after exercise.
- Extrasystoles – usually disappear with exercise when benign.
- Atrial flutter with variable block.

Abnormal pulse volume:

- Small, due to low cardiac output, e.g. severe cardiac failure/aortic stenosis (anacrotic pulse).
- Cardiogenic shock – the pulse pressure is small.

Large volume pulse:

- High cardiac output state, e.g. persistent ductus arteriosus.
- Aortic incompetence.
- Thyrotoxicosis.
- Paget's disease.
- Also in elderly patients with low diastolic pressure due to arteriosclerosis. In all these conditions, the pulse pressure is high with diastolic often less than half the systolic pressure.

Pulsus bisferans:

- Mixed aortic valve disease

Jerky pulse:

- HOCM

Examination of apex beat. The apex beat is not easily palpable due to obesity, breast tissue in females, emphysema, etc. Left ventricular hypertrophy causes a forceful localized apex beat and during examination the finger is lifted during systole. When such an impulse is displaced, the left ventricle is also dilated. The apex beat is also displaced to the left due to scoliosis of the spine and lung pathology. A double impulse apex beat is felt in HOCM.

A right ventricular impulse (right ventricular heave) is best felt by placing the hand left of the sternum. It is pronounced in right ventricular hypertrophy but is easily palpable in patients with a thin chest wall. In obese patients or in the presence of emphysema, the right ventricular impulse is often absent and may not be felt even in the presence of hypertrophy. In severe pulmonary hypertension the pulmonary impulse is palpable in the second left intercostal space and the forceful closure of the pulmonary valve is easily felt.

A thrill is a palpatory component of a murmur and is only palpable when the murmur is loud.

Auscultation of the heart sounds. The phonocardiogram reveals four normal components: mitral valve closure (M1), tricuspid component (T1), aortic component (A2), pulmonary closure (P2).

The first heart sound is caused by closure of mitral and tricuspid valves in that order. It is loud due to a tachycardia or in mitral stenosis. A decreased intensity of the first heart sound is due to a low cardiac output state or mitral incompetence.

Varying intensity of the first heart sound is due to complete heart block or atrial fibrillation.

The second heart sound is caused by closure of aortic and pulmonary valves in that order. The two components are easily audible in children and young adults and is called split second sound. In older adults the two components are close together and do not sound split. Th aortic component of the second heart sound is loud in hypertension and faint or absent in calcific aortic stenosis. The pulmonary component is loud in pulmonary hypertension and faint in Fallot's tetralogy. Unlike aortic stenosis, the pulmonary component is easily audible in pulmonary stenosis.

Splitting of the second sound is wide due to a right bundle branch block; splitting is paradoxical in left bundle branch block and severe aortic stenosis and fixed in secundum ASD.

The fourth sound is due to atrial contraction just after the 'p' wave in the electrocardiogram. The atrial sound is heard in hypertensive heart disease or as a gallop in left ventricular failure. The gallop rhythm is also audible due to accentuated third heart sound in patients with left ventricular failure. Third heart sound is audible in VSD, severe mitral incompetence, in childhood and in pregnancy. An opening snap is an extra sound heard in the earlier part of diastole in mitral stenosis.

Ejection clicks are due to a jet of blood causing vibration in a dilated aorta or pulmonary artery. A pulmonary ejection click is best heard at the left sternal edge, accentuates during inspiration and is heard invalvar pulmonary stenosis, idiopathic dilatation of pulmonary artery and in severe pulmonary hypertension.

The aortic ejection click is best heard near the apex during expiration and is heard in valvar aortic stenosis and dilatation of ascending aorta (e.g. aneurysm, Fallot's tetralogy/pulmonary atresia, coarctation of aorta, bicuspid aortic valve). A late ejection systolic click is heard in mitral valve prolapse and is often followed by an ejection systolic murmur.

Cardiac murmurs occur during systole or diastole. A systolic murmur is not always pathological, but the diastolic murmurs are mostly due to valvar abnormality.

Systolic murmurs are of two types: pan-systolic and ejection systolic.

Pan-systolic murmurs are due to flow of blood from higher pressure to a relatively low pressure cardiac chamber. There is no crescendo. The murmur starts at the first heart sound and occupies the full period of systole. For example, in mitral incompetence, this is best heard at the apex and radiates towards the axilla. The pan-systolic murmur of a VSD is heard at the left lower sternal edge. The murmur of tricuspid incompetence is similar to the VSD and is invariably due to dilatation of the right ventricle with presence of congestive cardiac failure with accentuation during inspiration. A late ejection systolic murmur is seen in mitral valve prolapse.

Ejection systolic murmurs have a crescendo–descrescendo sound and often fill only part of systole. The murmur of aortic stenosis is best heard in the aortic area but also in the lower left sternal and apical regions. The ejection murmur of pulmonary stenosis (P.S) is best heard in the pulmonary area, where a longer murmur signifies a more severe lesion. A secundum ASD has a similar murmur as in PS but is usually softer with fixed splitting of the second sound.

Insignificant systolic murmurs may be physiological as in pregnancy or during exercise, or due to causes such as aortic sclerosis (second sound easily audible) and murmurs transmitted from lower common carotid bruit.

Diastolic murmurs are the mid-diastolic murmurs of mitral stenosis/tricuspid stenosis, or secondary to the increased flow seen in mitral incompetence/VSD. An early diastolic murmur is seen in aortic incompetence, pulmonary incompetence. Graham Steel murmur is heard at the left sternal region. This is due to severe pulmonary hypertension, resulting in pulmonary artery dilatation and the pulmonary second sound is loud. An Austin Flint mid-diastolic murmur in severe aortic incompetence is rare.

Continuous murmurs can be due to a venous hum (especially in children), persistent ductus arteriosus, excessive bronchial circulation (e.g. pulmonary atresia), pulmonary arteriovenous fistula, peripheral pulmonary artery stenosis (often heard in patients with rubella syndrome), rupture of sinus of valsalva in right ventricle and pericardial rubs.

Further reading

Badgett RG, Lucey CR, Mulrow CD. Can the clinical examination diagnose left-sided heart failure in adults? *Journal of the American Medical Association*, 1997; **277**: 1712–19.

ANTIARRHYTHMIC THERAPY

Antiarrhythmic drugs have been regularly used to treat cardiac arrhythmias in clinical practice, but the different drug classes have very different modes of actions and primary indications in management of the different cardiac arrhythmias.

There are currently two main systems, the traditional (and most widely used) one being the modified Vaughan–Williams classification which has been taught for the last 20 years or so, which is based on physiological principles and cellular electrophysiology in normal experimental animal heart tissues. A newer alternative classification, known as the Sicilian Gambit, is based upon the different antiarrhythmic agents incorporating likely arrhythmia mechanisms, drug effects, drug receptors as well as ion channels, and clinical consideration for the given drugs.

Nevertheless, antiarrhythmic drugs are used predominantly in the ischaemic and failing human heart. The different classifications may therefore fail to anticipate individual patient response in clinical practice. The dose of the optimal suppressive drug should therefore be titrated against response and possibly guided by plasma concentration. The temptation to use combination antiarrhythmic therapies remains problematic in the absence of expert assessment and should be avoided.

The modified Vaughan–Williams classification

The Vaughan–Williams classification is based on the broad effects of antiarrhythmic drugs on ECG intervals, focusing generally on electrophysiological properties on each agent. The basic system was defined using transmembrane action potentials on myocytes of normal animal tissue. Nevertheless, this classification is widely used in everyday clinical practice, when referring to the different drugs.

The Vaughan–Williams classification has some limitations in each antiarrhythmic drug, has multiple actions at different concentrations, and different effects depending on the nature of the underlying cardiac rhythm. There are also some drugs which can belong to more than one Vaughan–Williams class. For example amiodarone can have properties of all four classes, whilst sotalol has both Class II (beta-blocker) and Class III properties. In addition, the beneficial effect of some drugs cannot be purely ascribed to its primary Vaughan–Williams electrophysiological class, as mechanisms linking anti-arrhythmic drug action to Vaughan–Williams class and to the mechanisms of arrhythmogenesis and clinical effectiveness are not clear. There are also reservations regarding the relationship of experimental and experimentally based classification to clinical application especially in diseased human hearts. The CAST (Cardiac Arrhythmia Suppression Trial) illustrates these concerns where the adverse effects of antiarrhythmic drug (mainly Class I) treatment were not predicted by the different drug classifications.

Class I drugs. These are the agents which effect the voltage-dependent sodium channel. The subclassification is based upon the drug effects on cardiac action potential duration, with Class Ia drugs prolonging the action potential, Class Ib shortening it and Class Ic having little or no effects on the action potential duration.

Class Ia drugs have been in use for a long time for both supraventricular and ventricular arrhythmias, and typically include quinidine, procainamide and disopyramide. Nevertheless, these drugs have different individual pharmocokinetic properties, including differences in onset and duration of dose-related properties. For example, quinidine has marked anticholinergic effects; procainamide has an active metabolite (N-acetyl procainamide) which is metabolized differently depending on acetylator status (leading to lupus-like side effects) and has myocardial depressant effects; and disopyramide has some peripheral vasodilator activity. These drugs have a pro-arrhythmic effect, with prolongation of the QT interval, leading to polymorphic ventricular tachycardia (torsades des pointes).

Class Ib agents such as lignocaine, primarily act on ventricular arrhythmias. Lignocaine use is suggested in cardiac resuscitation guidelines for malignant ventricular arrhythmias, but is short acting and can be administered paraenterally only.

Class Ic agents, such as flecainide, encainide and propafenone, act on both supraventricular and ventricular arrhythmias. The use of these agents in patients with structural heart disease, especially poor left ventricular function or severe ischaemic heart disease, has been associated with an adverse outcome. Recent evidence suggests that Class Ic agents (flecainide and propafenone) are effective agents for supraventricular arrhythmias, especially paroxysmal atrial fibrillation, cardioversion of atrial fibrillation and maintenance of sinus rhythm post-cardioversion.

Class II drugs. This refers to agents with sympatholytic activity, primarily the beta-adrenergic receptor blocking drugs. They include the non-selective lipophilic drugs (propranolol), drugs with high intrinsic sympathomimetic activity (pindolol) and the beta-selective drugs, such as metoprolol and atenolol.

Class III drugs. These drugs prolong the repolarization phase of the action potential, and are used for the treatment of both supraventricular and ventricular arrhythmias. Examples include sotalol, amiodarone and bretylium. Sotalol is frequently used in clinical practice, in view of its good tolerability and effectiveness, as evidenced by the recent ESVEM trial. Amiodarone is commonly used in patients with structural heart disease, especially in those with poor left ventricular function, as it probably has the least negative inotropism. Recent trials of amiodarone in left ventricular impairment have reported both positive (GESICA) and negative results, in reduction of mortality and morbidity. Two trials (EMIAT and CAMIAT) using amiodarone post-myocardial infarction did not confer any significant mortality advantage. Bretylium is used intravenously for cardioversion of ventricular arrhythmias, but is limited by severe hypotension.

Class IV drugs. This incorporates the calcium antagonist effects of verapamil and diltiazem, where there are effects on the conducting tissues of the heart, particularly at the atrio–ventricular node. These agents are used for supraventricular arrhythmias only, for example, the treatment and prophylaxis of supraventricular tachycardia, or in controlling the ventricular response to atrial fibrillation.

The Sicilian gambit

The actions of antiarrhythmic drugs are complex at the cellular level which makes their classification a complex issue. This has lead to a new classification, called the Sicilian Gambit, which identifies each antiarrhythmic drug by the primary site of action in the treatment of an arrhythmia. The mechanism for an arrhythmia can be defined, the electrophysiological property whose modification is likely to suppress the arrhythmia identified, the responsible ion current or receptor mediating that modification is stated, and the drug enacting the desired change can therefore be selected and dose titrated. The Sicilian Gambit is therefore an alternative system of classification based on the individualized origin of arrhythmia in the patient, which has its proponents, but its use in clinical practice is still not widespread.

Further reading

CAST Investigators. Effect of encainide and flecainide on mortality in a randomized trial of arrhythmia supression after myocardial infarction. *New England Journal of Medicine,* 1982; **321:** 406–12.

Harrison DC. The Sicilian Gambit – reasons for maintaining the present anti-arrhythmic drug classification. *Cardiovascular Research,* 1992; **26:** 566–7.

Rosen MR for the European Working Group on Arrhythmias. The Sicilian Gambit: a new approach to the classification of anti arrhythmic drugs based on their actions on arrhythmogenic mechanisms. *European Heart Journal,* 1991; **12:** 1112–31.

ANTITHROMBOTIC THERAPY IN CARDIOVASCULAR DISORDERS

Warfarin

Warfarin is the most widely used oral anticoagulant in Britain, although other oral anticoagulants such as Phenidione and Nicoumalone are available they are less commonly used. The antithrombotic effects of warfarin reflect its anticoagulant effects, which are mediated through its ability to inhibit thrombin generation by reducing levels of four vitamin-K-dependent coagulation factors (Factors II, VII, IX and X). Owing to this mechanism of action, warfarin can take 48–72 hours for the anticoagulant effect to develop fully and if an immediate anticoagulant effect is required, heparin must be used concurrently.

Indications

Oral anticoagulants have been shown to be effective in the following situations: (i) the primary and secondary prevention of venous thromboembolism; (ii) the prevention of stroke and systemic embolism in patients with tissue and mechanical prosthetic heart valves or with atrial fibrillation; (iii) the prevention of acute myocardial infarction (MI) in patients with peripheral arterial disease; and (iv) the prevention of stroke, recurrent infarction and death in selected patients following acute myocardial infarction. For most indications, an anticoagulant effect with a target International Normalized Ratio (INR) of 2.0–3.0 is appropriate. However, higher intensity anticoagulation with a target INR of 3.0–4.5 is used in patients with mechanical prosthetic heart valves.

1. Prevention of venous thromboembolism. Oral anticoagulants are effective in preventing venous thrombosis and pulmonary thromboembolism after hip surgery and major gynaecological surgery, and in patients with recurrent venous thromboembolism.

2. Treatment of deep vein thrombosis. Oral anticoagulant treatment is required for 3 months or more in patients with proximal (i.e. 'above knee') venous thrombosis and after 3 months in patients with symptomatic calf vein thrombosis.

3. Prosthetic heart valves. Clinical trials have confirmed the effectiveness of warfarin in this group of patients compared to aspirin-containing anti-platelet drug regimens. Warfarin is necessary in metallic valves (aiming for a target INR of 3.0–4.5) but in bioprosthetic valves, aspirin may suffice in low-risk patients.

4. Atrial fibrillation. Warfarin reduces the risk of stroke in atrial fibrillation by two-thirds. Patients with particular high risk are those aged >75 years; and those <75 years with risk factors such as hypertension, heart failure, previous stroke or transient ischaemic attack, diabetes and episodes of systemic thromboembolism. The recommended therapeutic range is an INR of 2.0–3.0, except in higher risk patients.

5. Acute myocardial infarction. Moderate-dose warfarin therapy aiming for an INR of 2.0–3.0 is effective in preventing stroke and venous thromboembolism in selected patients following acute myocardial infarction. High risk patients include those with dilated poorly contracting ventricles, and those with aneurysms, valve disease, atrial fibrillation or previous thromboembolism.

Interactions

The dose response to warfarin is influenced by both pharmacokinetic factors (due to differences in absorption or metabolism of warfarin) and pharmacodynamic factors (due to the intrinsic differences in patient response to warfarin doses). Hereditary resistance to warfarin has also been described where patients require warfarin doses that are 5–24 times higher than average.

1. Drugs. These can influence the pharmacokinetics of warfarin by reducing the absorption from the gut or altering its metabolic clearance. Changes in the patient's condition, particularly through intercurrent illness and drug administration necessitate more frequent testing of the anticoagulant effect. Major changes in diet, especially involving vegetables and alcohol consumption, may also influence warfarin control. Examples of drug interactions are as follows:

- Impaired absorption, hence reducing warfarin effect, e.g. cholestyramine.
- Enhancement of effect by drugs that inhibit metabolic clearance of warfarin, e.g. phenylbutazone, sulphinpyrazone, antibiotics (such as metronidzole, septrin), amiodorone.
- Inhibition of metabolic clearance by inducing activity of hepatic enzymes, hence inhibition of warfarin effect, e.g. barbiturates, carbamazepine, long-term alcohol use.
- The anticoagulation effect of warfarin is augmented by cephlosporins due to inhibition of vitamin K metabolism.
- Excess thyroxine increases the rate of metabolism of coagulation factors, potentiating warfarin.

2. Other interactions with warfarin. Some fluctations of vitamin K intake occur in both apparently healthy and sick subjects, affecting anticoagulation control. For example, increased intake of dietary vitamin K may occur in patients on weight reduction diets which are rich in green vegetables. Conversely, the effects of warfarin can be potentiated in patients with poor vitamin K intake, especially if concurrent treatment with antibiotics and intravenous fluids occurs or in malabsorption states. High metabolic states such as fever and hyperthyroidism increase responsiveness to warfarin.

3. Warfarin in pregnancy. Anticoagulants are teratogenic and should not normally be given in the first trimester of pregnancy. Women at risk of pregnancy should be warned of this danger. Warfarin also crosses the placenta with a risk of placental and foetal haemorrhage. Warfarin should, therefore, be avoided in pregnancy especially in the first and third trimesters.

4. Patients at increased risk of bleeding. Such patients include those with age >65 years, a history of uncontrolled hypertension (defined as systolic blood pressure >180 mmHg or diastolic blood pressure >100 mmHg), alcohol excess, liver disease, poor drug or clinic compliance, bleeding lesions (especially gastrointestinal blood loss, e.g. peptic ulcer disease, or recent cerebral haemorrhage), a bleeding tendency (including coagulation defects, thrombocytopenia) or concomitant use of non-steroidal anti-inflammatory drugs. The atrial fibrillation trials also suggested that instability of INR control and INR >3.0 were added risk factors for bleeding complications.

Aspirin

Aspirin is a useful antiplatelet agent, which acts by inhibition of cyclo-oxygenase. At low doses (75–300 mg/day), it inhibits prostacyclin (PGI_2), hence inhibiting platelets. At higher doses, aspirin may have effects on the thromboxane pathway, resulting in reduced thromboxane A2 synthesis and potentially, a vasoconstrictive effect.

Aspirin has been shown to be useful at a dose of 75–300 mg/day in: (i) secondary prevention of cardiac ischaemic syndromes, e.g. post MI or CABG, unstable angina, (ii) prophylaxis in moderate-risk patients with non-rheumatic atrial fibrillation, (iii) treatment of pre-eclampsia, (iv) prophylaxis against transient ischaemic attack and stroke, (v) reduction of thromboembolic events in patients with peripheral arterial disease. The recent International Stroke Trial and Chinese Acute Stroke Trial suggested that the use of aspirin in the acute period following ischaemic non-haemorrhagic stroke conferred a small benefit on stroke mortality. The Antiplatelet Trialists' Collaboration overview did not identify any significant differences in clinical outcome between the different doses of aspirin.

The main complications relating to aspirin use are related to gastrointestinal disturbances and allergy.

Ticlopidine and clopidogrel

Ticlopidine is a new thienopyridine derivative, which acts as an antiplatelet agent. It is useful for: (i) prevention of intracoronary stent thrombosis, and (ii) prophylaxis against stroke or transient ischaemic attack. Its efficacy is at least equivalent to aspirin, and may be useful in patients intolerant of aspirin. However, there is a 1% risk of developing pancytopenia and allergy.

Clopidogrel is chemically related to ticlopidine. Clopidogrel blocks activation of platelets by adenosine diphosphate (ADP) by selectively and irreversibly inhibiting the binding of this agonist to its receptor on platelets, therefore by affecting ADP-dependant activation of the glycoprotein (Gp)IIb–IIIa complex, the major receptor for fibrinogen which is present on the platelet surface.

In several experimental studies, clopidogrel prevents arterial as well as venous thrombosis and reduces atherogenesis. A recent randomized clinical trial (CAPRIE) to assess the potential benefit of clopidogrel, compared with aspirin in reducing the risk of ischaemic stroke, myocardial infarction or vascular death in patients with recent ischaemic stroke, recent myocardial infarction or peripheral vascular disease demonstrated that long-term administration of clopidogrel to patients with atherosclerotic vascular disease was more effective than aspirin in reducing the combined risk of ischaemic stroke, myocardial infarction or vascular death. The overall safety profile of clopidogrel was at least as good as that of medium-dose aspirin.

Dipyridamole

Dipyridamole is an antiplatelet agent, which works by the inhibition of phosphodiesterase, thereby preventing the degradation of cyclic AMP (cAMP) to AMP. The increased cAMP reduces platelet reactivity by decreasing platelet calcium and inhibiting PGI_2 synthesis.

Dipyridamole is commonly used for a variety of indications for its putative antiplatelet action, but there is insufficient evidence to support whether dipyridamole has any additional benefit to aspirin, e.g. in ischaemic heart disease, or maintaining long-term coronary artery bypass graft patency. The Second European Stroke Prevention Study (ESPS2) suggested that aspirin plus dipyridamole is useful as thromboprophylaxis against stroke or transient ischaemic attack, with an efficacy exceeding either agent alone.

The only licensed indication for dipyridamole is its use as an adjunct to oral anticoagulation for thromboembolism associated with prosthetic heart valves. Dipyridamole is useful as a pharmacological stress agent, in the diagnosis of ischaemic heart disease using radionuclide imaging (e.g. a dipyridamole thallium scan).

Heparin

Heparin potentiates antithrombin III activity, and therefore inhibits the instrinsic coagulation pathway. Heparin can be administered subcutaneously or intravenously, and lower low molecular weight isoforms have been shown to demonstrate greater half-life and clinical efficacy.

Subcutaneous heparin is useful in the following clinical indications: (i) prophylaxis against deep venous thrombosis and pulmonary thromboembolism (at a dose of 5000 iU b.d. or t.i.d.), (ii) prophylaxis against mural thrombus in patients following anterior myocardial infarction (at a dose of 12 500 iU b.d.), (iii) unstable angina (using low molecular weight heparin). The recent International Stroke Trial and Chinese Acute Stroke Trial suggested that the use of large subcutaneous heparin in acute stroke had a beneficial effect on stroke recurrence, but this was offset by increased haemorrhagic transformation, resulting in no overall benefit on stroke mortality. The recent ESSENCE and FRIC trials have suggested that low molecular weight heparin is useful in unstable angina.

Intravenous heparin is useful in the following situations: (i) early treatment of venous thrombosis and thromboembolism, and atrial fibrillation, while oral anticoagulation with warfarin is being introduced; (ii) unstable angina, in combination with aspirin.

The majority of problems relating to heparin use are bleeding, thrombocytopenia and osteoporosis.

Other antithrombotic agents

Thrombolytic agents such as streptokinase and tissue plasminogen activator (tPA) have now been well-established in the treatment of acute myocardial infarction, and will be discussed in a later topic. tPA has also been licensed for use in the USA for the treatment of acute thrombotic stroke in patients presenting within 3 hours of ictus onset. Studies of thrombolytic agents in acute stroke have generally been disappointing, with most trials demonstrating an excess of mortality and bleeding in the treated groups; nevertheless, one study has shown a reduction in disability (but not mortality) in stroke patients presenting early (within 3 hours) and who were treated with tPA.

Other antithrombotic agents, such as hirudin and GpIIb–IIIa inhibitors (ReoPro) show great promise in the treatment of unstable angina and as an adjunct to coronary angioplasty or stent.

Further reading

Antiplatelet Trialists' Collaboration. Collaborative overview of randomised trials of antiplatelet therapy–I. Prevention of death, myocardial infarction and stroke by prologed antiplatelet therapy in various categories of patients. *British Medical Journal,* 1994; **308:** 81–106.

Dalen JE, Hirsh J (ed.). Fourth American College of Chest Physicians Consensus Conference on Antithrombotic Therapy. *Chest,* 1995; **108** (4): Supplement.

Gibbs CR, Lip GYH. Do we still need dipyridamole? *British Journal of Clinical Pharmacology,* 1998; in press.

Related topics of interest

AORTIC DISEASE

The aorta begins at the aortic valve and runs initially cephalad (the ascending aorta), turns postero-laterally to the left (transverse arch), then caudally to pierce the diaphragm (descending thoracic), and finally passes through the posterior abdomen immediately anterior to the lumbar spine, ending at the level of L4 (abdominal aorta) with the bifurcation into the common iliac arteries. The aorta can be affected by disorders causing narrowing (occlusive disorders) or dilatation (aneurysms).

Occlusive disorders of the aorta

1. Atherosclerosis. This is the most common cause of aortic occlusive disease and affects mainly the lower abdominal aorta, where it causes ischaemia of the legs. This will be described in the topic 'Peripheral Vascular Disease'. Atherosclerosis can affect the whole aorta and if the aortic wall is diseased at the site of origin of a major artery, the organ which that artery supplies may become ischaemic. The most common organs to be affected in this way are the gut and kidneys.

(a) Chronic gut ischaemia (mesenteric angina) is rare and only happens when two of the three vessels supplying the gut (coeliac axis, superior mesenteric and inferior mesenteric arteries) are diseased. Presentation is usually with severe post-prandial pain and weight loss.

(b) Renal artery stenosis presents with uncontrolled hypertension with deteriorating renal function or renal failure especially if bilateral and may be exacerbated by the use of angiotensin converting enzyme (ACE) inhibitors. Definitive diagnosis rests on angiography and treatment can be by percutaneous angioplasty or direct surgical reconstruction.

2. Coarctation of the aorta. This occurs in 1 in 16 000 births and is usually found near the site of the ligamentum arteriosum. Rarer forms affect the ascending aorta or the upper abdominal aorta causing renal artery stenosis. There may be associated patent ductus arteriosus or other congenital cardiac defects, such as bicuspid aortic valve. The most common presentation is in early adult life with hypertension (often asymptomatic) or lower limb symptoms, and can include headaches, fatigue or intermittent claudication. Some patients develop rare complications such as heart failure (especially children), endocarditis, aortic dissection, aneurysm formation or cerebral haemorrhage. Hypertension due to coarctation of the aorta is often due to a combination of mechanical and renal factors, with activation of the renin angiotensin system. Physical examination reveals radiofemoral delay and a systolic murmur audible over the spine. The chest X-ray shows rib-notching. Diagnosis can be confirmed by aortography and treatment commonly is by percutaneous balloon angioplasty, with surgery being reserved for resistant, recurrent cases or those with associated anomalies. It is well recognized that hypertension often persists in up to one-third of patients despite successful correction of coarctation. Persistence of hypertension following correction may be related to the duration of prior hypertension, and vasomotor changes, including structural alterations, and increased vascular resistance or reactivity in the upper part of the body.

3. Aortic dissection. Aortic dissection occurs from an intimal tear that allows the passage of blood into the media, creating a false channel contained externally by the outer adventitial layers of the aorta. With each systolic pulse the shear stresses generated extend the dissection either proximally or distally potentially leading to cardiac tamponade, aortic regurgitation, aortic rupture or branch artery compromise. Tears involving the ascending aorta are known as Stanford type A (DeBakey I–II) and those involving the descending aorta beyond the subclavian artery Stanford type B (DeBakey III) dissections. In DeBakey Type I the ascending and descending aorta are involved, while in Type II there is involvement of the ascending aorta only. Type III involves the descending aorta only, which is the most favourable type prognostically.

Typically dissection presents with a sudden, severe or tearing, retrosternal chest pain which radiates posteriorly to the interscapular region or the base of the neck. Signs may include aortic regurgitation, a difference in blood pressure between the two arms, absent pulses or evidence of haemorrhage. The condition may also present with an acute abdomen, stroke or MI, and occasionally as hemiplegic or paraplegic (due to spinal artery involvement) or Horner's syndrome.

Predisposing factors are hypertension, cystic medial necrosis and Marfan's syndrome. The majority of patients are male around the sixth decade but pregnant women can also be affected.

Indications for surgery

Type I and II cases must always be referred urgently for surgical repair to a cardiac surgeon because of the overwhelming risk of fatal complications (50% will be dead within 48 hours) unless the patient has prohibitive risks of medical debility, extensive renal or bowel infarction or stroke when surgery may be deferred. Type III can be treated conservatively initially with controlled hypotension but should be referred for operation if patients have persistent pain, uncontrollable hypertension, aneurysmal expansion or rupture, or there is evidence of end organ ischaemia (spinal cord, kidneys, gut or legs).

Preoperative assessment

On suspicion of the diagnosis all patients should be treated pharmacologically to reduce the blood pressure to a systolic pressure of around 110 mmHg, heart rate to 60–70 bpm, and the force of systolic ejection. Beta blockade and sodium nitroprusside help smooth control. Patients should be nursed in the ITU with full invasive monitoring. Diagnostic tests are performed on an urgent basis and aimed at confirming the dissection, identifying whether the ascending aorta is involved and defining any vascular abnormalities resulting from the dissection.

Although the choice of the imaging techniques is dictated by their availability, the expertise and particular requirements at the time, all patients must have an electrocardiogram (ECG) and chest X-ray. The ECG may help exclude MI and will support the diagnosis of dissection if there are signs of left ventricular hypertrophy. In 80% of patients chest X-ray may show widening of the mediastinum, widened aorta, pleural effusion, cardiomegaly, disparity in size between ascending/descending aorta, changes is successive radiographs and displacement of calcified plaques (by 10 mm).

In acute situations urgent confirmation is required and echocardiography (transthoracic or transoesophageal), assists with diagnosis at the bedside. Pathognomic signs include demonstration of two channels, intimal flap or differential flow between the two channels. Diastolic fluttering of the anterior mitral leaflet and abnormal Doppler flow patterns in the left ventricular outflow tract in diastole may also indicate dissection. Computed tomography/magnetic resonance imaging (CT/MRI) scan, is useful for confirmation of the diagnosis. Aortography can identify the entry site and the extent of dissection. It is often preferable to transfer patients to a cardiothoracic centre after initial medical therapy and stabilization.

Surgical management

For type A dissection total cardiopulmonary bypass is instituted and the aortic root transected in order to inspect the aortic valve. Some patients may require aortic valve replacement or resuspension. Resection of the tear in the ascending aorta is followed by reapproximation of the aortic wall or replacement with an interposition Dacron graft. For tears located in the arch extensive surgery may be required when flow into the carotid and subclavian vessels has been severely compromised. For type B dissection, where operative mortality is 40% and survival no better than with careful medical management, the situation is less clear. Complications of bleeding, cerebral, visceral, lower limb ischaemia, renal artery compromise, persistence of pain, uncontrolled hypertension and progressive widening of the mediastinum or expanding distal aneurysm warrants surgical intervention. Repair involves resection of the intimal tear and interposition Dacron graft. If there is evidence of visceral artery compromise without rupture, aortic fenestration can be performed without grafting.

Prognosis	Careful long-term follow-up is required since 25% of patients will need one or more further operations and hypertension should be monitored. Serial non-invasive imaging techniques and assessment are especially important. Annually, 8% of patients will die most of them from cardiovascular complications.
Abnormal aortic aneurysms	Abnormal aortic aneurysms are common in the elderly (present in 2% of men >65 years of age) and are usually confined to the infrarenal aorta (>95%) but may extend distally to involve the iliac arteries. Aneurysms involving the renal and visceral artery origins or extending more proximally are relatively rare. The cause is generally atherosclerosis (smoking and hypertension are the usual risk factors) but 10% have a familial history with an affected first degree relative, and 10% are so called inflammatory aneurysms, which are characterized by pain, systemic disturbance and a raised erythrocyte sedimentation rate (ESR). The aetiology is largely unknown.

Presentation is most commonly with rupture and sudden death. Other presentations are as an incidental finding, abdominal or back pain, emboli, or the patient may have noticed the lump or a sensation of pulsation or his 'heart beating in the abdomen'. Ruptured aneurysm may present with the classical triad of severe abdominal and back pain, collapse and a palpable expansile abdominal mass. Eighty per cent of ruptured aneurysms result in sudden death, and of the remainder only 50% survive. Once the diagnosis is made immediate surgery is the only hope of survival. Time must not be wasted in organizing unnecessary investigations such as CT scan, chest X-rays, etc.

The best initial investigation of a suspected abdominal aneurysm is ultrasound. All aneurysms greater than 4 cm in diameter or causing symptoms must be referred to a vascular surgeon for consideration for operative repair. The patients general health, especially cardiac and respiratory and renal status, must be assessed carefully. The risk of rupture is proportional to the maximal diameter of the aneurysm and rises steeply in aneurysms greater than 5 cm diameter.

Further investigations may include CT scan to assess the upper and lower extent of the aneurysm and many surgeons now undertake radionuclide myocardial imaging and echocardiography to detect reversible ischaemic heart disease and assess cardiac function preoperatively. Appropriate therapy may reduce the operative risk and the detection of severe cardiac disease may influence the decision to repair a relatively small aneurysm (5–6 cm). Elective surgical repair by aneurysm resection and inlay Dacron grafting is well established and carries an operative mortality of <5% in most cases. Endovascular repair is currently an experimental procedure but may be of value in the future.

Repair of supra renal aneurysm is a more difficult procedure carrying risks of gut, renal and spinal cord ischaemia. This has a mortality approaching 20%, should generally be recommended only for fitter patients with large aneurysms and be carried out by surgeons with specific expertise in this area.

Further reading

Anagnostopoulos CE, Prabhakar MJS, Kittloe CF. Aortic dissections and aortic aneurysms. *American Journal of Cardiology,* 1972; **30:** 263–73.

de Giovanni J, Lip GYH, Osman K, Mohan M, Islim IF, Gupta J, *et al.* Percutaneous balloon dilatation of aortic coarctation in adults. *American Journal of Cardiology,* 1996; **77:** 435–9.

de Leeuw PW, Birkenhäger WH. Coarctation of the aorta. In: Swales JD, (ed.) *Textbook of Hypertension.* Oxford: Blackwell, 1994; 969–79.

Treasure T, Raphael MJ. Investigation of suspected dissection of the thoracic aorta. *Lancet,* 1991; **338:** 490–5.

Related topics of interest

Hypertension (p. 132)
Peripheral vascular disease (p. 167)

ARRHYTHMIAS – ATRIAL FIBRILLATION AND ATRIAL FLUTTER

Atrial fibrillation

Pathophysiology. During atrial fibrilation the atrial impulses discharge at a rate between 350 and 600/min, resulting in small, irregular 'f' (fibrillation) waves. As only occasional impulses penetrate the atrioventricular node, there is a totally irregular ventricular rhythm, which is the characteristic of this arrhythmia. Rapid atrial fibrillation with a rapid ventricular response may be easily mistaken for other supraventricular arrhythmias, for example, atrial flutter or supraventricular tachycardias. Variation in the R–R interval is the important clue.

The predominant problems associated with atrial fibrillation are haemodynamic and thromboembolic. Loss of atrial transport in atrial fibrillation can result in a reduction of stroke volume by 20–30%, especially in elderly subjects. Fast atrial fibrillation also results in an inefficent diastolic filling, leading to myocardial ischaemia and heart failure. These haemodynamic consequences result in the typical symptoms of dyspnoea and reduction in exercise tolerance, or heart failure. Furthermore, intra-atrial stasis contributes towards thrombus formation, particularly in the left atrial appendage. This is more likely in the presence of a dilated left atrium or poor left ventricular function, or any clinical risk factors (such as hypertension) and can result in stroke and thromboembolism. The risk of stroke in a patient with non-valvular atrial fibrillation is 5% per year, this figure increasing substantially (17-fold) if mitral valve disease is present.

Aetiology. The common aetiological factors associated with atrial fibrillation are hypertension, ischaemic heart disease, valve disease and thyroid disease. Hypertension accounts for up to 50% of atrial fibrillation in community studies, such as the Framingham study and the West Birmingham Atrial Fibriilation project. By contrast, ischaemic heart disease is the more common aetiological factor amongst patients with atrial fibrillation presenting to hospital. Thyroid disease is often unrecognised amongst patients with atrial fibrillation, especially in the elderly where the signs of thyrotoxicosis may be less obvious. However, atrial fibrillation may occur in the setting of any pyrexial illness, post-operatively (especially after thoracotomy), intra-thoracic pathology (lung tumours, pleural effusion, pulmonary thromboembolism, etc.) and in association with heart disease (for example, cardiomyopathy, conduction abnormalities such as the Wolff–Parkinson–White syndrome, atrial septal defect, etc). For example, atrial fibrillation can occur in ~20% of cases following coronary artery bypass surgery. Alcohol is another precipitating factor, and in some series, is said to account for up to two-thirds of new-onset atrial fibrillation in patients aged <65 years (holiday heart syndrome). Idiopathic or 'lone' atrial fibrillation is a diagnosis of exclusion, where subjects have no clinical aetiological factor, a normal ECG (apart from atrial fibrillation), a normal chest X-ray and a normal echocardiogram.

Clinical features. Atrial fibrillation is often asymptomatic. In the West Birmingham Atrial Fibrillation Project, only one-third of patients had ever been admitted to hospital. Others present with typical cardiorespiratory symptoms, such as dyspnoea, fatigue, syncope, chest pain, thromboembolism, etc. Atrial fibrillation is associated with heart failure in 30% (range 10–50%) and is present in 15% of ischaemic/thrombotic stroke patients. Nevertheless, atrial fibrillation has been reported in 11% of haemorrhagic stroke patients in the Oxfordshire Community Stroke Study.

Management. Management of atrial fibrillation requires documentation of the arrhythmia and possible aetiological or precipitating factors. Patients with paroxysmal atrial fibrillation need a careful history to ascertain the frequency and duration of symptoms. Such patients then need to be considered for antiarrhythmic therapy (to suppress paroxysms and to maintain sinus rhythm), and antithrombotic therapy. Suitable agents for paroxysmal atrial fibrillation include sotalol, Class 1 agents (propafenone, flecainide, etc - but not in poor left ventricular function), and amiodarone. Digoxin should not be used in paroxysmal atrial fibrillation as the evidence suggests that patients treated with digoxin have more frequent paroxysms and faster atrial fibrillation rates.

By contrast, treating chronic atrial fibrillation requires consideration of the objective of management, that is, either cardioversion to sinus rhythm or heart rate control. The long-term prognostic implications of either strategy still remain uncertain, and are being investigated in a large randomized study, the Atrial Fibrillation Follow-up Investigation of Rhythm Management (AFFIRM).

If elective cardioversion to sinus rhythm is the primary objective, patients invariably need anticoagulation with warfarin for 3 weeks prior to cardioversion and for at least 4 weeks post-cardioversion. In emergency cardioversion, patients should be started on intravenous heparin pre-cardioversion and warfarin for 4 weeks post-cardioversion. Methods of cardioversion can be either pharmacological (using Class I or III, with an average success rate of ~75%) or electrical (by synchronized direct current shock, with an immediate success rate of ~90%). Digoxin has no value whatsoever in cardioversion of atrial fibrillation nor the long-term maintenance of sinus rhythm. Apart from anticoagulation post-cardioversion, consideration is needed for antiarrhythmic drug use to maintain sinus rhythm; without such drugs only 29% remain in sinus rhythm at 1 year follow-up. Predictors of successful cardioversion and maintenance of sinus rhythm include age, prior duration of atrial fibrillation (lower success if duration >12 months), presence of structural heart disease (including mitral valve disease, valve prosthesis,etc), lack of obvious precipitating factor which has been corrected (such as chest infection, thyroid disease pyrexial illness), etc.

If atrial fibrillation rate control is the primary objective, consideration of antiarrhythmic and anticoagulation drugs is needed. Digoxin is the commonest drug prescribed for rate control, although it is increasingly less so in North America. Digoxin is useful in controlling the resting heart rate in atrial fibrillation, but is of limited value in exercise or in conditions of high cathecholamines (for example, post-operatively, post-thoracotomy), acute on chronic heart failure, etc. In such cases, rate control may necessitate other agents such as beta-blockers, calcium antagonists (verapamil, diltiazem) or amiodarone.

Anticoagulation of atrial fibrillation has been addressed by many recent large-scale randomized trials, and the available evidence suggests that warfarin reduces the risk of stroke in nonrheumatic atrial fibrillation by two-thirds. Warfarin is definitely indicated in patients with atrial fibrillation and previous cerebrovascular events, structural heart disease (dilated atria, poor left ventricular function) or clinical risk factors (such as age >75 years, hypertension, heart failure, diabetes, etc). A relative indication is paroxysmal atrial fibrillation, and such patients should be warfarinized if they have frequent paroxysms and any evidence of structural heart disease. Young patients (age <60 years) with lone atrial fibrillation are considered to be at low risk of thromboembolism and are unlikely to need warfarin. The efficacy of aspirin is less certain, but the evidence suggests that it may be useful in low risk patients with atrial fibrillation, with the overall reduction in stroke risk by 21%.

Based upon clinical criteria, most patients with AF can be classified into high, moderate and low risk patients (*Figure 1*):

- High risk patients (annual risk 8–12%) with AF should be started on warfarin (target INR 2.0–3.0, reduces annual risk to 1–4%); if

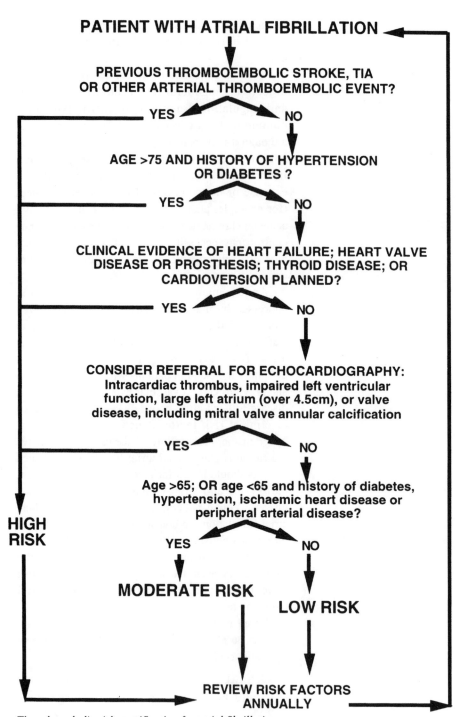

Thromboembolic risk stratification for atrial fibrillation

contraindications to warfarin exist (such as bleeding, falls, compliance, concomitant diseases), aspirin 75–300 mg/day should be prescribed.
- Moderate risk patients (annual risk 4%) with atrial fibrillation should be started on either warfarin (target INR 2.0–3.0, reduces annual risk to 1–2%) OR ASPIRIN 75–300 mg/day (reduces annual risk to 1–2%) – in this group, it is less certain for the superiority of warfarin over aspirin, therefore individual circumstances have to be considered.
- Low risk patients (annual risk 1%) should receive aspirin 75–300 mg/day if possible.
- If contraindications to both warfarin and aspirin exist (particularly gastrointestinal bleeding, allergy, etc), this should be carefully documented in clinical notes and in cases of uncertainty, specialist cardiology referral is suggested.

Risk stratification should be reviewed at regular intervals, and at least annually.

Further reading

Atrial Fibrillation Investigators. Risk factors for stroke and efficacy of antithrombotic therapy in atrial fibrillation. Analysis of pooled data from five randomized controlled trials. *Arch. Intern. Med.* 1994; **154:** 1449–57.

Atrial Fibrillation Investigators. The efficacy of aspirin in patients with atrial fibrillation. *Arch. Intern. Med.* 1997; **157:** 1237–40.

The AFFIRM Investigators. Atrial Fibrillation Follow-up Investigation of Rhythm Management - the AFFIRM Study Design. *Am. J. Cardiol.* 1997; **79:** 1198–1202.

Lip GYH, Golding DJ, Nazir M, Beevers DG, Child DL, Fletcher RI. A survey of atrial fibrillation in general practice: The West Birmingham Atrial Fibrillation Project. *Br. J. Gen. Pract.* 1997; **47:** 285–89.

Lip GYH, Lowe GDO. ABC of Atrial Fibrillation. Antithrombotic treatment for atrial fibrillation. *Br. Med. J.* 1996; *312:* 45–9.

Atrial flutter

Pathophysiology. In atrial flutter there is a re-entrant circuit within the atria, resulting in the atria discharging at a rate of appproximately 300/minute. Most commonly, the circuit lies within the right atrium, and is conducted along the lateral right atrium and 'returns' superiorly along the atrial septum. Atrial discharges result in the characteristic 'F' or flutter waves, resulting in a saw-tooth pattern, which are best seen in leads II, III and aVF, or V1. The conducting ability of the atrioventricular node determines the ventricular response. Most commonly, alternate atrial impulses are conducted to the ventricles, resulting in a ventricular rate close to 150/min (that is, atrial flutter with 2:1 block). Nevertheless, variable atriaoventricular block can result in an irregularly irregular rhythm, mimicking atrial fibrillation.

Clinical features and management. Many of the aetiological factors and clinical features are common to both atrial flutter and atrial fibrillation. Nevertheless, management strategies differ. Atrial flutter with variable atrioventricular block is commonly confused with atrial fibrillation.

The most effective treatment of atrial flutter is synchronized direct current electrical cardioversion, which is successful in >90% of cases. Low energy defibrillation may suffice, for example, starting at 25–50 J. Primary drug treatment of atrial flutter is less successful, but atrial flutter sometimes degenerates into atrial fibrillation, which is easier to treat pharmacologically then atrial flutter. Commonly used drugs, which act at the atrioventricular node, such as digoxin, adenosine, verapamil and quinidine, occasionally convert atrial flutter to atrial fibrillation or result in a higher degree of atrioventricular block (for example, 3:1 or 4:1). By contrast, the use of a Class I agent (for example, quinidine, disopyramide) in patients with atrial flutter may accelerate the ventricular response with a 1:1 atrioventricular conduction. This may be due in part to the slowing in atrial rate and the anticholinergic effects (especially with disopyramide and quinidine) which result in an increase in atrioventricular conduction. With atrial flutter it is therefore advisable to administer Class I agents with digoxin, beta-blocker or verapamil to avoid the potential for the accelerated atrioventricular conduction.

Patients with atrial flutter who undergo elective cardioversion should be anticoagulated in a similar manner to atrial fibrillation. Electrical cardioversion is far superior to pharmacological cardioversion, the latter usually having an efficacy rate of approximately 25–30% with conventional Class Ic and Class III agents. A recently introduced Class III agent, ibutilide, reports a conversion rate of 42% for atrial flutter, and has been licensed for such use in the United States of America.

ARRHYTHMIAS – BRADYARRHYTHMIAS

This is often the result of failure of cardiac impulse formation or conduction.

Sinus bradycardia

Defined as sinus rhythm at <60 beats per minute, may occur in patients with no underlying heart disease (physiological), including those with hypothermia, hypothyroidism, hyperkalaemia, in the context of acute myocardial infarction or in association with certain drugs such as digitalis, or the commonly used beta-adrenergic blocking agents. The latter can also include the eye drops for glaucoma.

Sick sinus syndrome

This is common in the elderly and manifests a wide spectrum of bradyarrhythmias and atrial tachyarrhythmias, including paroxysmal atrial fibrillation. Some patients exhibit persistent or intermittent sinus or nodal bradyarrhythmias which may alternate with supraventricular tacharrhythmias, the so-called the brady-tachy syndrome.

The ECG shows sinus pauses or sinus arrest for longer than 2 seconds during the waking hours; such pauses are accepted during sleeping periods or in the presence of atrial fibrillation.

Permanent pacemaker implantation should be considered for patients with symptomatic bradycardias or those in whom antiarrhythmic therapy of atrial arrhythmias can only be given safely with pacemaker support.

Atrio-ventricular (AV) conduction abnormalities

First degree AV block. This is characterized by a prolonged P-R interval (from the beginning of the P wave to the beginning of the QRS complex) of more than 200 msec. It can be due to increased vagal tone in some normal individuals or caused by digitalis, beta blockers, myocarditis, diptheria and some forms of congenital heart disease. Patients are usually asymptomatic and no therapy is needed.

Second degree AV block. Mobitz type I or Wenckebach phenomenon reflects conduction problems in the AV node, and refers to consecutively conducted impulses with progressively prolonged P-R intervals until the P wave is not followed by a QRS complex. It is usually asymptomatic, common in subjects with high vagal tone (e.g. sleep, athletes), and is not progressive and does not affect long-term prognosis. However, symptomatic cases may need to be considered for pacing, as in a patient with syncope it may reflect serious AV conduction disorders.

Mobitz type II AV block reflects conduction problems in the His–Purkinje system, and refers to consecutively conducted impulses with normal P-R intervals associated with sudden failure of impulse conduction. This reflects a serious conduction system disorder and often progresses to complete heart block (CHB). Permanent pacing is indicated.

Third degree AV block (CHB). This is characterized by AV dissociation and a slow idioventricular rhythm.

Congenital CHB is frequently asymptomatic and associated with a heart rate of 45–65/min with narrow QRS complexes. If the heart rate increases with exercise, no further therapy is needed. If associated with structural or congenital heart abnormalities, if wide QRS complexes are present, or if the 24 h Holter monitor shows junctional exit block, paroxysmal tachycardia or a daytime junctional rate of <50/min, then permanent pacing is indicated.

In acquired CHB, the heart rate is usually 20–50/min and associated with a wide QRS complex. It is often due to idiopathic degeneration of the conducting fibres without other cardiac pathology (Lenegre's disease), although acute CHB can occur in acute myocardial infarction. The patient may present with lightheadedness, giddiness, syncope, transient amnesia, exercise intolerance, or worsening heart failure. Occasionally patients with suspected epilepsy or transient ischaemic attacks are shown to have intermittent CHB as the cause of

Management of bradyarrhythmias

symptoms. Permanent pacing is indicated and improves long-term outlook.

In the emergency situation as in collapse or shock, an intravenous injection of atropine and isoprenaline infusion should be given, or external cardiac pacing attempted, whilst preparing for temporary transvenous demand pacing.

Patients with symptomatic sinus node disease, Mobitz Type II AV block or complete heart block are normally considered for permanent pacemaker implantation. In the context of an inferior myocardial infarction, conduction disorders usually recover within 2–3 weeks; with anterior MI, prognosis is determined by LV dysfunction and co-existing ventricular arrhythmias.

Related topic of interest

Pacemakers (p. 163)

ARRHYTHMIAS – SUPRAVENTRICULAR

Atrial ectopic beats

These are a common occurrence, and may account for an 'irregular pulse', leading to the erroneous diagnosis of atrial fibrillation. Multifocal atrial ectopics are particularly common in pulmonary disease. Long pauses may follow as sinus node automacity is depressed by the ectopic beat. They are generally asymptomatic, and there is little need for antiarrhythmic therapy.

Sinus tachycardia

This is defined as sinus rhythm at a greater rate than 100 beats/min. Characteristically, sinus tachycardia has a gradual onset and termination. P waves (best seen in leads II or V1) precede each QRS complex. In cases of apparent sinus tachycardia at rest, it is also important to exclude atrial tachycardia or atrial flutter.

Sinus tachycardia is often physiological, that is, in response to stress, anxiety, exertion, etc. Nevertheless, sinus tachycardia at rest may be due to thyrotoxicosis fever or alcohol excess.

Supraventricular tachycardias

There are many classifications of supraventricular arrhythmias. A simplified classification of supraventricular arrhythmias is as follows:

1. Atrial fibrillation.
2. Atrial flutter.
3. Supraventricular tachycardias.

- Atrial tachycardias.
- Junctional tachycardias – these are commonly divided into: (a) atrioventricular nodal re-entry tachycardias (AVNRT), with a micro-reentry circuit within the atrioventricular node. (b) atrioventricular re-entry tachycardias (AVRT), with bypass tract present (e.g. Wolff–Parkinson–White syndrome, Lown–Ganong–Levine syndrome).

Apart from atrial fibrillation and atrial flutter (which are usually classified and managed differently), other supraventricular arrhythmias are commonly regarded as 'supraventricular tachycardias'. The arrhythmia commonly referred to as a 'paroxysmal supraventricular tachycardia' (PSVT) in clinical practice usually refers to an atrioventricular re-entrant tachycardia. Symptomatic patients may be referred for electrophysical testing and possible ablation therapy if a bypass tract is present.

Therapy for supraventricular tachycardia usually consists of: (i) vagotonic manoeuvres, such as the Valsalva manoeuvre, carotid sinus massage; (ii) drugs acting at the atrioventricular node such as adenosine or verapamil, if a bypass tract is present; verapamil may accelerate conduction down the abberant pathway and should be used with caution; (iii) Class Ic (flecainide, propafenone) and Class III agents (sotalol, amiodarone) may be useful alternatives. Digoxin is useful in AVNRT.

Rapid atrial pacing (directly or via oesophagus) or DC cardioversion may be needed when medical therapy fails to terminate a tachycardia. In patients with abnormal conducting pathways (e.g. Wolff–Parkinson–White syndrome), ablation of the abnormal tract can be undertaken using radiofrequency ablation.

Atrial tachycardia

Atrial tachycardia is commonly confused with atrial flutter or fast atrial fibrillation. The main difference from atrial flutter is that the atrial rate is slower in atrial tachycardia, at 120–250/min. Atrial tachycardia has no saw-toothed appearance, and is due to an ectopic focus separate from the sinoatrial node. Abnormally shaped P waves best seen in lead V1 are at a regular rate, between 120 and 250/min. The QRS complexes are narrow, unless pre-existing conduction defect exists.

This arrhythmia is relatively uncommon, accounting for around 10% of supraventricular tachycardias. Atrioventricular block may co-exist. Paroxysmal atrial tachycardia with block is commonly associated with digoxin toxicity.

Junctional tachycardias

Atrioventricular nodal re-entry tachycardia (AVNRT). This requires the presence of a micro re-entry circuit within the atrioventricular node. The common form has a re-entry circuit with a slow antegrade limb and a fast retrograde limb to the re-entry circuit. The typical ECG shows the P wave buried in the QRS complex.

Atrioventricular re-entrant tachycardia(AVRT). This requires the presence of an accessory pathway remote from the atrioventricular node, providing a second connection between atria and ventricles. The arrhythmia therefore results from the repeated circulation of an electrical impluse between atria and ventricles. This is usually conducted from the atria to ventricle via the atrioventricular node (slowly), and then re-enters the atria via the (fast) additional pathway. Structural heart disease is usually absent

The ventricular response is regular, with atrial activity seen as inverted P wave, in the ST segment, after each QRS complex. QRS complexes are usually narrow and regular, at a rate of 130–250/min. Evidence of an accessory pathway on the surface ECG may be manifest as a short PR interval with (as in the Wolff–Parkinson–White syndrome) or without (as in the Lown–Ganong–Levine syndrome) a delta wave. Atrial fibrillation is a serious risk in these patients if the bypass tract is able to conduct rapidly. Syncope warrants urgent referral.

Sick sinus syndrome

This is a common condition, especially in the elderly, which is produced by idiopathic degeneration of the sino-atrial node, resulting in impaired sinus node function or sino-atrial conduction. The main problem is the development of bradycardias, for example, inappropriate sinus bradycardia or episodes of sinus arrest, sinus pauses or sinus exit block.

The sick sinus syndrome is often associated with a variety of atrial tachyarrhythmias, including atrial fibrillation, atrial flutter and atrial tachycardia, and its manifestations can range from asymptomatic to non-specific. These include dizziness, palpitations, fatigue, syncope and even sudden death. The use of drugs such as digoxin, beta-blockers and calcium antagonists may initiate or exacerbate symptoms in these patients.

The 'sick sinus' syndrome often becomes manifest after a paroxysm of tachycardia (where there is depression of sinus node automaticity) leading to sinus arrest or sinus bradycardia. In addition, an atrial tachyarrhythmia may start as an escape rhythm in the context of an underlying brady-arrhythmia, for example, sinus bradycardia or sinus arrest. Such alternation of tachycardias with bradycardias is commonly referred to as the 'tachy-brady' syndrome. Abnormal atrioventricular conduction may also co-exist in such patients.

It is therefore essential to consider this diagnosis before antiarrhythmic drug therapy or general anaesthesia in any patient with atrial fibrillation and a history of syncope or dizziness. In addition, if there is an underlying sick sinus syndrome, direct current (D.C.) cardioversion of atrial fibrillation may result in asystole and should be covered by a temporary pacemaker. Permanent pacemaker therapy (using an atrial or dual chamber system, depending on atrioventricular conduction) may be very successful in such patients, reducing arrhythmias, heart failure and improving prognosis.

Further reading

Zipes DP. Specific arrhythmias: Diagnosis and treatment. In: Braunwald E (ed.) *Heart Disease. A Textbook of Cardiovascular Medicine*, 4th Edn. Philadelphia: WB Saunders 1992; 667–25.

ARRHYTHMIAS – VENTRICULAR

Ventricular tachycardia

Definition. Three or more consecutive QRS complexes of ventricular origin (>0.125s) at a rate of 100–250/min.

Differential diagnosis. Supraventricular tachycardia with bundle branch block or aberrant ventricular conduction. The presence of AV dissociation, ventricular fusion or capture beats and identical ventricular extrasystoles during sinus rhythm (before or after) strongly favour the diagnosis of ventricular tachycardia.

Aetiology. The common causes are acute myocardial infarction, coronary artery disease and cardiomyopathy. It can also occur in valvular heart disease, particularly in aortic valvular disease, or be drug induced (digitalis toxicity, psychotropic drugs or a range of antiarrhythmic drugs), electrical accidents or related to electrolyte derangements, particularly low serum potassium, hypomagnesaemia or acid base imbalance.

Clinical significance. Ventricular tachycardia is often associated with a critical cardiac condition especially when the rate is 180–250/min. It may aggravate heart failure or shock. However, if it occurs at a slower rate (e.g. 120/min) or if left ventricular function is preserved it may well be tolerated. Prognosis depends on the symptoms. Fainting may reflect ventricular flutter or fibrillation and signals a high risk of sudden death. Prognosis may be good in the rare patient with no significant cardiac disease and without fainting.

Treatment of the acute attack. Intravenous bolus injection of lignocaine is given first followed by a DC synchronized shock if there is no response. Rhythm should be maintained by a lignocaine infusion afterwards. Other alternatives include intravenous beta blocker (especially after MI).

Amiodarone is particularly useful if left ventricular function is compromised. Intravenous amiodarone is increasingly used where other drugs fail. Other antiarrhythmic agents should be used cautiously in view of their potential for proarrhythmic effects (especially Class I agents) and the potential for negative inotropism (e.g. disopyrimide). If refractory overdrive pacing should be attempted. Drugs such as intravenous verapamil are contraindicated.

Long-term prophylaxis. Long-term prognosis in symptomatic VT may be poor and consideration should be given to early referral to an electrophysiology specialist if VT is recurrent. In the context of an acute MI prognosis may be reasonable and long term beta blocker treatment should be considered. An implantable anti-tachycardia pacemaker or defibrillator as well as electrical ablation of abnormal foci are experimental new approaches for the resistant patients. Resection of the arrhythmogenic area outlined by electrophysiological mapping and coronary artery bypass grafting might be an option in some cases.

Specific forms of ventricular tachycardia. Torsade de pointes: (twisting around a point) is polymorphic and usually non-sustained VT in which the axis twists giving rise to a sinusoidal appearance in the ECG. The QRS axis rotates 360° over a sequence of 5–20 complexes. The basic ECG may show QT prolongation, T-wave abnormalities or high amplitude U-waves of opposite polarity of the T-wave, reflecting the prolonged and widely dispersed repolarization process which is characteristic of the condition.

Causes of long QT intervals and *torsade de pointes* include congenital syndromes (Jervill–Lange–Nielsen or Romano–Ward syndromes), electrolyte imbalance (hypokalaemia, hypomagnesaemia, hypocalcaemia), drugs (class I, class III, phenothiazines, tricyclic antidepressants, antihistamines, macrolide antibiotics (erythromycin, clarithromycin)), poisons (organophosphates) and other conditions, such as AV block and bradycardia, cardiac ischaemia (myocardial infarction).

Correction of the electrolyte disturbance is often enough to treat torsade de pointes. Temporary pacing at a rate higher than sinus, isoprencline infusion are effective in the short term. In congenital long QT syndromes, beta blockers are beneficial. Suspected drugs should be withdrawn.

Effort induced ventricular tachycardia. This is one manifestation of the athletic heart syndrome, and the arrhythmia is often multifocal and preceded by ventricular multiple extrasystoles. It might also be caused by aortic stenosis, hypertrophic cardiomyopathy, ischaemic heart disease and mitral valve prolapse. Occasionally, however, no cause is found. Except in aortic stenosis, exercise testing should be performed to confirm the diagnosis, and this should be repeated after treatment with a beta blocker if there are no contraindications.

Ventricular tachycardia due to right ventricular dysplasia. Areas of the right ventricular outflow tract, often quite small, may be replaced by fat or fibrous tissue which act as a focus for a monomorphic ventricular tachycardia. This usually manifests in young individuals and shows a left bundle branch block pattern. Drugs or surgery are implemented as in case of non-specific ventricular tachycardia.

Fascicular tachycardia. It originates from the lower septum and shows a right bundle branch block pattern with left axis deviation. This is the one ventricular arrhythmia which is sensitive to adenosine and calcium antagonists, such as verapamil.

Cardiomyopathy-associated ventricular tachycardia. It often responds favourably to amiodarone but not other drugs.

Accelerated idioventricular rhythm (slow ventricular tachycardia). The ventricular rate is 60–110/min with competition with the sinus rhythm. Fusion beats are seen at the transition from one to the other. This arrhythmia usually occurs in myocarditis, acute myocardial infarction and digoxin toxicity. Treatment is rarely required but if the patient is haemodynamically compromised increasing the heart rate with atropine or atrial pacing suppresses the rhythm.

Ventricular flutter

Definition. It is a broad complex tachycardia with ventricular rate 250–300/min.

The individual components of the QRS complexes cannot be identified and they form a continuous undulating line.

Differential diagnosis. Atrial flutter with a 1:1 or 2:1 AV conduction ratio and aberrant conduction particularly in patients with WPW syndrome. Carotid massage may disclose flutter atrial activity or continuous monitoring may show dropout of QRS complexes revealing atrial flutter activity.

Aetiology. Similar to ventricular fibrillation.

Clinical significance. The rhythm may result in Stokes–Adams attacks if it is brief. It may deteriorate to ventricular fibrillation and cause sudden death.

Management. Similar to ventricular fibrillation.

Ventricular fibrillation

Definition. The QRST complexes are replaced by a fibrillatory line with continuous very rapid irregular deflections which may be fine, coarse or changing from one to another. It results in loss of consciousness and absence of palpable arterial pulse. It may be preceded by ventricular tachycardia or flutter, and commonly triggered by a ventricular extrasystole manifesting the R on T phenomenon.

Differential diagnosis. Ventricular arrest secondary to AV block or electromechanical dissociation due to cardiac rupture, massive pulmonary embolism, extensive myocardial infarction and sudden excessive blood loss.

Aetiology. Myocardial infarction and electrical instability (often compounded by electrolyte disturbances or drugs) are the commonest causes of ventricular fibrillation. Other causes include cardiomyopathy, valvular lesions, long QT syndromes and pre-excitation. Non-cardiac factors are similar to those causing ventricular tachycardia.

Clinical significance. The onset of ventricular fibrillation is followed by Stokes–Adams attacks and loss of consciousness. If allowed to continue it leads to sudden death. Ventricular fibrillation is responsible for 3/4 of all sudden cardiac deaths.

Management

Treatment of acute attack in the monitored patient. Following basic life support measures (airway and starting CPR (cardiopulmonary resuscitation)) a precordial thump should be given if appropriate. If ventricular fibrillation (or pulseless VT) is diagnosed, defibrillation and CPR should be continued. During CPR adrenaline should be given every 3 minutes and consideration given to buffers (bicarbonate), antiarrhythmic therapy (lignocaine, betrylium) and atropine/pacing as necessary.

Calcium salts are especially effective in hyperkalaemic patients, but should be avoided if hypokalaemia or digitalis intoxication are suspected. Temporary pacing is required if ventricular fibrillation developed from *torsade de pointes*.

Current Resuscitation Guidelines of the Resuscitation Council (UK) and European Resuscitation Council should be applied.

Treatment in the non-monitored patient. The patient has to be resuscitated and ventricular fibrillation has to be suspected. The same measures have to be followed until a cardiac monitor is obtained and other causes ruled out.

Prophylaxis in paroxysmal ventricular fibrillation. Prophylaxis for episodes occurring on a chronic basis with longer time intervals of days,weeks or months is the same as for ventricular tachycardia with more emphasis towards considering the implantable automatic cardioverter-defibrillator (ICD).This device is of the size of the first generation pacemakers and it is designed for patients with pharmacologically and surgically intractable paroxysmal ventricular tachycardia and fibrillation.

One electrode (rectangular in shape) is incorporated over the cardiac apex and the other electrode (which senses changes in cardiac rhythm and subsequently discharges 10–25 J when detecting ventricular tachycardia or fibrillation) is attached to a catheter, inserted through the superior vena cava, which is connected to the device. Recently a right ventricular catheter electrode, like that deployed for ventricular pacing, has been tried to discharge only 0.5–1 J which successfully converted ventricular tachycardia and fibrillation.

Further reading

Rankin AC. Non-sedating antihistamines and cardiac arrhythmia. *Lancet*, 1997; **350:** 1115–16.

```
┌─────────────────────────────────┐
│        BASIC LIFE SUPPORT       │
│                                 │
│   Check responsiveness, call for help │
│            open airway          │
│       check breathing, pulse    │
│            start CPR            │
└─────────────────────────────────┘
                 │
                 ▼
      Precordial thump (if appropriate)
                 │
                 ▼
       Attach defibrillator-monitor
                 │
                 ▼
            Assess rhythm
                 │
                 ▼
             Check pulse
```

VF pulseless VT	Non VF/VT
Defibrillate ×3 as necessary	
CPR 1 min	CPR up to 3 mins

During CPR: 1. Check electrode/paddle, positions/contact
2. Attempt intubation, IV access
3. Give adrenaline every 3 mins
4. Correct reversible causes*
5. Consider (i)   buffers (sodium bicarbonate)
          (ii) antiarrythmics (lignocaine etc.)
          (iii) atropine
          (iv) pacing

*Potentially reversible causes:
Hypoxia, Hypovolaemia, Hyper/hypokalaemia and metabolic disorders, Hypothermia,
Tension pneumothorax, Tamponade, Toxic/therapeutic disturbances,
Thromboembolic/mechanical obstruction

Flow diagram based on the 1997 Adult Advanced Life Support Guidelines of the
Resuscitation Council (UK)

CARDIAC FAILURE

Definition   Decrease in cardiac output, due to abnormality in structure and function of heart, leading to inability to meet the demands of the body.

Aetiology
- Abnormal myocardial function due to coronary artery disease, cardiomyopathy or myocardial infarction.
- Valvar disease: (a) pressure overload (aortic stenosis, aortic coarctation, pulmonary stenosis); (b) volume overload (aortic and mitral incompetence).
- Congenital heart disease (increased preload VSD, PDA).
- Systemic and pulmonary hypertension (elevated afterload on ventricles).
- Secondary to cor pulmonale (right ventricular failure).
- Excessive blood transfusion (increased preload).
- Increased metabolic demand: thyrotoxicosis, severe anaemia.

NB: In such 'high output' cardiac failure, although cardiac output is higher than average, it is *low* for the individual and insufficient to meet (increased) metabolic demands.

Types
- Left-sided failure, mostly due to ventricular dysfunction and valvar disease (including mitral stenosis) left ventricular myxoma, VSD and persistent ductus arteriosus.
- Combined, usually left-sided giving rise to right (congestive heart failure).

NB: Congestive heart failure is usually due to *systolic* malfunction of the ventricles, i.e. their inability to contract effectively. *Diastolic* dysfunction (failure to relax effectively) occurs in some hypertrophic and stiff ventricles in hypertensive heart disease and hypertrophic cardiomyopathy and infiltrative disease, e.g. amyloidosis, constrictive pericarditis and eosinophilic heart disease.

Pure diastolic dysfunction is uncommon and is usually seen in the elderly with hypertension or coronary arterial disease. In most cases there is mixed systolic and diastolic dysfunction, mostly seen in ischaemic heart disease and later stages of hypertrophic cardiomyopathy, untreated coarctation and aortic stenosis.

Epidemiology

The incidence of cardiac failure is increasing due to the increasing elderly population. The incidence of heart failure increases with age. Approximately 5% of hospital admissions are with cardiac failure. The incidence is higher in men as compared to women. The most common aetiological factors are hypertension, ischaemic heart disease (including myocardial infarction), valve disease, cardiomyopathy, etc. Alcoholic heart muscle disease, vitamin deficiencies (beri-beri) and drugs (cytotoxics) are unusual causes which should not be forgotten.

Classification

This is based on exercise capacity (the New York Heart Association — NYHA) classification.

1. Class I. No limitation in physical activity in the presence of cardiac pathology. This can only be suspected if there is history of cardiac disease and confirmed by investigators, e.g. echocardiography.

2. Class II. Slight limitation in physical activity only. More strenuous activity only causes shortness of breath, e.g. walking on steep inclines and several flights of steps. This group continues to have an almost normal lifestyle and employment.

3. Class III. More marked limitaiton of activity interfering with work. Walking on the flat produces symptoms.

4. Class IV. Breathless at rest and mostly house-bound.

Prognosis

Is worse in Class III and IV. Most long-term (10-year follow-up approximately) studies have been done before ACE inhibitors were widely used. In the Framingham study (1971) survival at 8 years in Class I to IV was 30%. Mortality in Class IV at 1 year was in excess of 60% and, in Class III and IV taken together, about 34% at 1 year. The prognosis usually depends on severity, age and sex (more in males).

Pathophysiology

Starling's original descriptions of cardiac function showed that an increased filling pressure in the left ventricle was associated with an increase in cardiac output. Increased venous return to ventricles, either from systemic (into the right atrium) or pulmonary (into the left atrium), is described as an increased *preload* and Starling's theory was that increased preload, increased the cardiac output. However, in diseased ventricles, this phenomenon is deficient. Also, rapid and excessive increase in preload in some normal patients can cause pump failure, e.g. over transfusion with intravenous infusions.

Afterload is the term used for pressure against which ventricles have to pump blood in systemic or pulmonary circulation. It is higher in systemic and pulmonary hypertension and usually associated with increased vascular resistance.

Compensatory mechanisms in cardiac failure

Lower cardiac output (stroke volume) provokes compensatory increase in heart rate mediated by adregenic system which improves the circulation. Diuretics in the early phases, in most patients, improve the symptoms, however, decreased blood volume often activates the sympathetic nerves and renin angiotensin aldosterone system. There is also activation of atrial naturetic factor (ANF) which attempts to cause some vasodilatation and diuresis. Prostaglandins (PGE2 and PGI2) are also elevated to restore vascular tone.

The venoconstriction and increased volume overload due to aldosterone results in higher preload and there is also an increase in arterial vasoconstriction (resistance) and afterload. This increased pre- and afterload which puts more burden on the failing ventricle and causes deterioration in cardiac failure.

Summary

Poor ventricular function
↓
Cardiac failure
↓
Decreased stroke volume
↓
Neurohumoral response: activation of
sympathetic/renin angiotensin aldosterone system
↓
Venoconstriction (increased preload);
vasoconstriction (increased afterload); fluid
retention; in some cases inappropriate tachycardia
↓
Further stress on ventricular wall and dilation
leading to worsening of ventricular function

Symptoms, signs, diagnosis

The main presenting symptom is shortness of breath, reduced exercise tolerance and fatigue. In more severe cases, the patient may complain of inability to lie flat (orthopnoea) and waking at night with shortness of breath (paroxysmal nocturnal dyspnoea). With these symptoms left-sided failure should be suspected. Swelling of ankles and feet is another common presenting feature, however, the common cause of this symptom is venous insufficiency, where the oedema is more pronounced in the evenings and usually disappears in the mornings.

Physical signs

(a) Left-sided failure:

- Orthopnoea.
- LV mostly dilated or hypertrophied or both.
- Crepitations and rhonchi.
- Third or fourth heart sound, termed 'gallop', in the presence of tachycardia.
- Pulsus alternans.

(b) Right-sided failure:

- Oedema (mostly absent in infants).
- Elevated jugular venous pressure (JVP).
- Hepatomegaly.

(c) Combined failure:

- Signs of both left and right heart failure.

Diagnosis
- Valsalva manoeuvre is absent.
- *Chest X-ray.* In most cases cardiac enlargement. In left-sided failure pulmonary venous congestion. This may be mild with upper lobe diversion or very severe with butterfly appearance in lungs. In acute left ventricular failure (e.g. acute myocardial infarction, acute valve regurgitation or acquired VSD) there may not be any enlargement of the heart. Only pulmonary congestion is noted.
- *ECG.* Is abnormal in the majority of adults and elderly patients. May be normal in exceptional cases, e.g. congenital, valvar disease, restrictive or early dilated cardiomyopathy.
- *Echocardiograms.* Impaired ventricular function or excessively hypertrophied wall of ventricles with diastolic dysfunction.
- *Cardiac catheterization, angiography and myocardial biopsy.* This is helpful in more difficult cases, e.g. restrictive and infiltrative cardiomyopathies and myocarditis (biopsy) and pericardial disease causing failure. Left ventricular angiography shows impaired function and elevated end-diastolic pressure.
- *24-hour ECG (Holter) monitoring.* In more severe cases ventricular extrasystoles, sustained or non-sustained ventricular tachycardia and abnormal atrial rhythms (extrasystole, supraventricular tachycardia and paroxysmal atrial fibrillation) are seen.

Exercise testing in cardiac failure
Exercise tolerance, when judged by treadmill or bicycle ergometry, is reduced. This test is not carried out in clinical practice but is useful when judging the effect of new drugs. In some cases, respiratory physiological measurements are made during exercise. Oxygen and CO_2 measurements and ventilation are estimated. Oxygen uptake (vO_2) and carbon dioxide production (vCO_2) are useful in checking the severity of failure. vO_2 uptake is

diminished. The maximum oxygen uptake (vO_{2max}) is defined as the value when vO_2 remains static in spite of increasing exercise and represents the upper limit of aerobic exercise tolerance.

Urea and electrolytes

In mild and moderate heart failure, renal function and electrolytes are usually normal. In Class IV heart failure, however, partly due to diuretics and sodium restriction, there is an inability to excrete water and dilution hyponatraemia is often seen. Vasopressin levels also contribute to this phenomenon. Potassium levels are usually normal but may be low when large amounts of diuretics are used without potassium supplementation or when patient's diet is poor (elderly). Hyperkalaemia can occur in severe congestive heart failure with low glomerular filtration rate, especially when patients are on large does of ACE inhibitors and potassium sparing diuretics are not discontinued. Low magnesium levels can occur with chronic treatment and may provoke ventricular tachycardia.

Renal blood flow and glomerular filtration decrease in cardiac failure. Proteinuria is a common feature. Though blood urea may be high, serum creatinine is usually normal in the absence of known renal disease. However, increasing serum creatinine levels, reflecting deteriorating renal function, may occur, especially in patients on large doses of diuretics and ACE inhibitor. In some cases, heart failure improves clinically with a decrease in the JVP and oedema with high blood urea and normal or slightly elevated serum creatinine. This picutre indicates dehydration due to excessive diuresis.

Liver function

In severe chronic congestive cardiac failure (CCF) with enlarged liver, function tests are abnormal with increased serum bilirubin, aspartate and lactate dehydrogenase levels.

Treatment of heart failure

Treatment is directed towards improving symptoms and prognosis. It depends on severity and type of failure and, to some extent, the cause.

1. Acute left ventricular failure
- Prop up the patient.
- Oxygen administration.
- Intravenous diamorphine.
- Consider intravenous nitrates, later switch to oral. Intravenous sodium nitroprusside can be used in acute VSD and mitral incompetence.
- Digoxin not helpful unless atrial fibrillation is present.

2. Chronic left ventricular failure
- Diuretics.
- Angiotensin converting enzymes (ACE) inhibitors.
- If ACE inhibitors cannot be tolerated, e.g. symptomatic hypotension or cough, consider oral isosorbide mononitrate and hydralazine up to 175 mg per day.

3. Congestive cardiac failure (severe)
- Bed-rest until signs and symptoms improve. This decreases the metabolic demand and increases the renal perfusion provoking diuresis.
- Salt intake must be reduced – avoid added salt and salty food.
- In more severe cases, intravenous diuretics, e.g. frusemide or with added metolazone 2.5–10 mg per day.
- Vasodilators: ACE inhibitors alone or in combination with oral nitrates and hydralazine.
- Digoxin may have some benefit in reducing heart failure admissions, but not mortality.
- Intravenous inotropes, such as dopamine and dobutamine, may be useful in hypotension and heart failure. Inotropes may also serve as a bridge to cardiac transplant or corrective valve surgery.

Special surgical procedures Cardiac transplantation (patients aged preferably under 58–60 years). Intra-aortic balloon couterpulsation and left ventricular assist devices are used as bridges to cardiac transplantation or before coronary artery bypass surgery in the presence of poor cardiac function.

Closure of VSD secondary to acute myocardial infarction and mitral regurgitation secondary to ruptured chordeatendinae. Rarely, resection of large ventricular aneurysms, if combined with coronary bypass surgery, is helpful.

Heart failure with atrial fibrillation

Digoxin

Digoxin used in the presence of artrial fibrillation (AF) improves both failure (inotropic effect) and slows heart rate allowing effective filling of the ventricle. In acute LV failure, without AF, there is no evidence that digoxin is helpful but in chronic failure in sinus rhythm there is some evidence that it may be of help. The dose depends on age and renal function. Rapid digitalization orally or intravenously (when orally restricted, e.g. post-operative) is seldom required. However, in rapid AF compromising haemodynamics, loading doses of 1–1.75 mg can be given over a period of about 24 hours, usually divided into two to three doses.

The maintenance dose varies from 125 to 500 μm a day and is less in the elderly or renally impaired. Intravenous dose is about 60–75% of the oral dose. In mild renal impairment reduced doses should be used and digoxin levels monitored (6 hours after the previous dose should be between 1.2 and 1.9 ng/ml).

Potassium levels should be checked — low potassium levels provoke arrhythmias. These include ventricular extrasystoles, atrioventricular (AV) junctional rhythms and nodal or atrial tachycardia. Even ventricular tachycardia (VT) can occur. Pauses due to sinus block, Wenckebach second degree AV block can also occur. ST segment sagging in ECG is often seen and does not indicate toxicity.

Nausea, vomiting and headaches, confusion, visual symptoms like halos and changes in colour perception, and gynaecomastia are not uncommon. Serious toxicity should be treated by correction of potassium levels and drugs, e.g. beta blockers, or by glycoside-binding agents like cholestyramine. Specific antibodies have been used but are expensive and not freely available.

Anticoagulants

These should always be considered if atrial fibrillation is present. In patients in sinus rhythm, especially when the left atrium and ventricle are considerably dilated, the incidence of thromboembolism is higher, especially in patients with dilated cardiomyopathy and where the ejection fraction is less than 25%.

ACE inhibitors

Various large scale studies like *CONSENSUS I* have shown that ACE inhibitors, besides improving symptoms, also considerably improve prognosis. The action of ACE inhibitors is through arteriolar and venous dilatation. However, sudden deaths that occur in heart failure are not reduced.

ACE inhibitors are also useful in cardiac dysfunction and failure after acture myocardial infarction.

Beta blockers in CHF

The concept of using beta blockers in heart failure is not new. However, they are not widely used. One theory is that they reduce inappropriate tachycardia induced by excessive catecholamine secretion. Also, they may, by their negative inotropic effect, protect against the damaging effect of catecholamines on the myocardium and dangerous arrhythmias. Recently, carvedilol, which has both beta- and alpha-blocking properties, has shown encouraging results in residant cases. This drug has also been used after acute MI to improve prognosis.

Alpha blockers (e.g. prazosin) have been used in the past. They are not widely used now because of the development of tolerance.

Rehabilitation

In controlled chronic heart failure, excessive rest should not be advised, since this may cause loss of muscle mass in the lower limbs and possibly vasoconstriction and further disability. Patients should be encouraged to go out for walks but should know their limits. Excessive fatigue or breathlessness should be avoided. Graduated

exercise has been shown to improve cardiac
performance by enhancing oxygen uptake.

Further reading

Dargie HJ, McMurray JVV. Diagnosis and management of heart failure. *British Medical Journal*, 1994; **308:** 321–8.

Lip GYH, Sarwar S, Ahmed I, Lee S, Kapoor V, Child D, Fletcher I, Cox I, Beevers DG. A survey of heart failure in general practice. The West Birmingham Heart Failure Project. *European Journal of General Practice*, 1997; **3:** 85–9.

Lip GYH, Zarifis J. Diastolic dysfunction: a review. *European Journal of Internal Medicine*, 1995; **6:** 145–54.

Related topic of interest

Ischaemic heart disease – myocardial infarction (p. 154)

CARDIAC SURGERY – VALVULAR HEART SURGERY

In the developed world with a decline in rheumatic heart disease, ischaemic and degenerative valve disease in an ageing population are the prevalent causes of much of the morbidity and mortality associated with acquired valvular heart disease. Congenital valve problems, e.g. bicuspid aortic valve, may not manifest until adulthood.

Diseased atrioventricular valves, namely the mitral and tricuspid valves, and the semilunar valves, that is, the aortic and pulmonary valves, may be stenosed or regurgitant although there may be an element of both problems. In stenosis the cardiac chamber proximal to the valve hypertrophies to generate enough force to maintain an adequate output. Regurgitation, on the other hand, produces volume load and results in a combination of dilatation and hypertrophy of the proximal chamber. In general, regurgitation is better tolerated than stenosis.

Generally patients with acquired valvular heart disease present when an asymptomatic murmur is detected on routine examination. Dyspnoea and poor exercise tolerance are common symptoms although the clinical picture depends very much on the type of valve involved. A careful history and thorough physical examination, including dental assessment, are made. ECG may show a hypertrophied heart chamber, arrhythmias or evidence of ischaemia. A chest X-ray may reveal enlargement of the cardiac chambers and great vessels and the condition of the lung fields.

Echocardiography is the first line of investigation for the assessment of patients. It is extremely valuable as a non-invasive procedure suitable for serial assessment of cardiac function and valve motion/pathology. In addition to ventricular wall thickness, motion and chamber dilation, two-dimensional and M-mode assessment may demonstrate valve thickness, motion or calcification. Doppler flow helps estimate the gradient across a stenotic valve and the presence of regurgitation, although this may be semi-quantitative.

Angiography confirms the echocardiographic findings and becomes essential in patients aged over 50 years for identification of co-existing coronary artery disease.

Indications for surgery

1. Aortic stenosis. Although surgery is generally not indicated in the asymptomatic patient a majority of patients with critical stenosis (area <0.75 cm^2) will become symptomatic in a short period. The indications for surgery are the presence of angina, CHF or syncope. Surgery should be performed before left ventricular failure occurs since the patient is at real risk of sudden death. Symptoms are usually associated with an area of <0.8 cm² and a transvalvular peak gradient of >50 mmHg. However, as the left ventricular function deteriorates, a gradient of 30 mmHg may be sufficient indication for surgery.

2. Aortic regurgitation. Although minor degrees of aortic regurgitation are well tolerated chronic regurgitation produces pressure and volume overload of the left ventricle with progressive ventricular dilation and failure and surgery should be performed sooner. Acute regurgitation results in acute left ventricular failure and pulmonary oedema. The left ventricular end-systolic dimension (LVESD), measured by echocardiography is a useful guide and if the LVESD is greater than 55 mm left ventricular dysfunction may be irretrievable. Indications for surgery are acute aortic regurgitation with failure; endocarditis with haemodynamic compromise, persistent sepsis, or recurrent systemic embolization; symptoms of angina or congestive heart failure; or evidence of left ventricular decompensation in the asymptomatic patient with ejection fraction of <45%, or LVESD approaching 55 mm by echocardiography.

3. Mitral stenosis. This occurs almost exclusively as a result of rheumatic fever and may be mimicked by left atrial myxoma or thrombus. Surgery is indicated for patients with severe symptoms (NYHA III–IV) pulmonary hypertension or a resting pressure gradient of 10 mmHg across the mitral valve, or NYHA II when the critical valve area of <1 cm² is present. Systemic embolization from a left atrial thrombus despite adequate anticoagulation is another indication for surgery. The patient requires medical stabilization before surgery which includes correction of fluid overload and anticoagulation. Mitral valvotomy is often successful in competant non-calcified valves, however mitral valve replacement may be necessary in patients with valvular calcification. The aim of surgery is to enlarge the orifice and restore function. A pliant, mobile valve may benefit from balloon valvulotomy, which is a safe and efficient procedure but restenosis is likely and replacement may be required.

4. Mitral regurgitation. Although it is difficult to be precise about indications for operation since patients with similar haemodynamics may have different symptoms, definite indications include acute regurgitation associated with CHF or cardiogenic shock; acute endocarditis; NYHA class III–IV symptoms; class I–II symptoms with evidence of deteriorating left ventricular function, that is, an ejection fraction of <55%, or LVESD approaching 50 mm by echocardiography. Transoesophageal echocardiography provides improved assessment of valve function. However, the valve can be properly assessed only at operation and repaired under direct vision. Increasingly successful repair and valve conservation is utilized but some are not suitable for repair and require replacement.

Surgical valve replacement or repair?

Aortic valves are generally replaced since reparative techniques have not shown long-term durability. For mitral valves a variety of repair techniques is available and the majority of non-rheumatic mitral valves are amenable to repair. The choice of procedure is based primarily on the anatomical and functional involvement of each valve that can be accurately determined preoperatively. Assessment involves a study of the valve complex; the annulus, leaflets, chords and papillary muscles, and the pathology. Each structure may be normal, restricted or have increased mobility or a combination. A stenotic valve with good pliability will be suited for commissurotomy. A regurgitant valve with only a dilated annulus will be perfect for a straightforward repair. Valve with chordal/papillary muscle elongation or rupture requires a more complex reconstruction while a completely destroyed valve with severe fibrosis/calcification will require replacement. If reconstruction is difficult then the benefits of repair may be marginal compared to replacement.

Prosthetic valves

Apart from closed mitral valvotomy all valve operations are performed under direct vision on cardiopulmonary bypass and consist of excising and replacing the valve with a *biological* or *mechanical* prosthesis. Bioprostheses may be *heterografts*, composed either of porcine valves or bovine pericardial tissue mounted on a frame, or *homografts*, which are preserved human valves. Mechanical valves composed of metal or carbon alloy are classed according to their structure as caged-ball, single tilting disk or bileaflet tilting disk valves. Prosthetic valves differ from one another with regard to durability, thrombogenecity and haemodynamic profile. Between 10 and 20% of homografts and 30% of heterografts fail within 10–15 years particularly in patients under 40 years of age, and require replacement. With rare exceptions mechanical valves are very durable lasting 20–30 years.

Mechanical valves are thrombogenic and patients require life-long anticoagulant therapy with an IMR around 3.0. Bioprostheses have a low thrombogenic potential hence, long-term anticoagulation is not usually required. Each prosthetic valve has its own haemodynamic profile and effective orifice area. Heterografts have the largest effective orifice area, similar to that of a native valve. Porcine valves and caged-ball valve types have the smallest effective orifice area and are therefore potentially obstructive.

Based on the above characteristics mechanical valves are preferred in young patients, those who have a life expectancy of more than 10–15 years, or those who require long-term anticoagulant therapy for other reasons, e.g. atrial fibrillation. Bioprostheses are preferred in the elderly, those with a life expectancy of less than 10 years, or who cannot (or will not) take long-term anticoagulant therapy. The selection of valve suitable for the needs of the patient is at times difficult and is often helped by involving the patient in the decision-making. All patients with biological or mechanical valves are at risk of endocarditis.

Results of surgery

Mortality of elective aortic valve replacement is low. Stroke, arrhythmia and bleeding account for 1–2% of hospital deaths although mortality increases with age, poor left ventricular function or emergency replacement. The 5-year survival is 85% which is much better than that of untreated symptomatic aortic stenosis. Benefits in terms of survival for regurgitation may be marginal for aortic regurgitation.

The mortality of mitral valve surgery, due especially to increased mitral repairs, has steadily declined although for mitral valve replacement has not fallen below 5%. Pulmonary hypertension, right ventricular failure, long-standing mitral valve disease and increased patient age all add to the surgical risk. The risk is lowest in rheumatic heart disease and highest in those with ischaemic heart disease. The 5-year survival is around 80% and 10-year survival is 60%.

Complications of prosthetic valves

There are a number of problems associated with prosthetic valves, which may be technical and related to the valve itself or a result of valve replacement in general. Valve-related complications are thromboembolism, haemorrhage, structural valve failure, non-structural dysfunction, prosthetic endocarditis and valve-related mortality.

1. Thromboembolism. Thrombus tends to form on artificial valves and may embolize with consequent morbidity and mortality. Although mechanical valves are more thrombogenic than tissue valves, with adequate anticoagulation the frequencies of valve thrombosis and systemic embolization are similar for both types. Risk of thromboembolism is higher for implants at the mitral site, for multiple prosthetic valves, for patients in atrial fibrillation, aged over 70 years and with depressed left ventricular function.

2. Bleeding episodes. Patients receiving anticoagulants are at a greater risk from bleeding episodes. This risk is higher in the elderly. Short-term control over anticoagulant is managed with fresh frozen plasma. Vitamin K may be used to reverse anticoagulation but makes further management difficult due to its prolonged effect on the synthesis of clotting factors.

3. Valve failure. In general structural failure in mechanical valves is rare but when it occurs it is sudden and often has catastrophic haemodynamic consequences. About 30% of heterografts and 10–20% of homografts fail progressively with time and may be replaced electively. Paravalvular leak between the suture ring and the annulus is commonly a technical problem although prosthetic endocarditis may also cause a paraprosthetic leak. Consequent haemodynamic problems or haemolytic anaemia necessitates further surgery.

4. Prosthetic valve endocarditis. All patients are at risk of prosthetic valve endocarditis which occurs in 3–6% of patients. Prophylactic antibiotics must be given before any dental or surgical procedure. Fever is the most common symptom, a new or changing murmur, systemic embolization, haemodynamic changes or CHF are present in 30–70% of patients. The focus of infection is often the suture ring. Early diagnosis with repeated blood cultures is essential and despite high-dose antibiotics, the mortality from this complication is over 20%. Surgery is best deferred until the infection is under control, but continued sepsis, haemodynamic instability or systemic embolization warrants early operation.

Related topics of interest

Cardiovascular investigations – cardiac catheterization (p. 85)
Infective endocarditis (p. 140)

CARDIAC SURGERY – CORONARY ARTERY SURGERY

Ischaemic heart disease is a major cause of morbidity and mortality in developed countries and results from an imbalance of oxygen supply and demand resulting in inadequate myocardial perfusion to meet metabolic demands (ischaemia). Coronary artery disease may be asymptomatic, until it presents as sudden death or an acute MI or symptomatic. In patients with coronary artery disease coronary revascularization is undertaken for symptomatic relief and/or prognostic benefit (*Table 1*) and can be by balloon angioplasty with or without stenting or by surgery, i.e. coronary artery bypass grafting.

Table 1. Indications for coronary revascularization

Symptomatic relief

1. Class III–IV chronic stable angina refractory to medical therapy.
2. Unstable angina refractory to medical therapy, in whom PTCA is unlikely to relieve ischaemia.
3. Acute ischaemia or haemodynamic compromise following percutaneous transluminal coronary angioplasty (PTCA).
4. Acute evolving infarction within 4–6 hours of the onset of chest pain, not suitable for PTCA.
5. Ischaemic pulmonary oedema.
6. Markedly positive stress test before major intra-abdominal or vascular surgery.

Prognostic benefit

1. Left main stenosis >50%.
2. Triple vessel disease with impaired ejection fraction.
3. Triple vessel disease with significant inducible angina.
4. One- and/or two-vessel disease with extensive myocardium in jeopardy but lesion not amenable to PTCA.

Miscellaneous

1. Anomalous coronary artery with risk of sudden death.
2. Postinfarction mechanical defects (ventricular aneurysm, septal rupture, acute mitral regurgitation).

Symptomatic relief

Symptomatic coronary disease is initially treated pharmacologically with nitrates, beta-receptor blocking agents and/or calcium antagonists. However, patients with refractory angina or in whom the degree of ischaemia, symptomatic or not, threatens to lead to MI are prime candidates for revascularization.

Prognostic benefit

Three large, prospective, randomized trials comparing medical therapy versus surgery have shown that patients with left main stem stenosis and severe triple vessel disease with impaired left ventricular function fare better with surgical revascularization than medical treatment. This group of patients includes those without disabling angina or refractory ischaemia in whom the extent of coronary disease, ventricular function and the degree of inducible ischaemia on stress testing are such that surgery may improve long-term survival by delaying infarction and preserving ventricular function.

Surgery is also indicated for rare anomalies of coronary arteries with risk of sudden death.

Assessment of the patient for surgery

Patients with ischaemic heart disease require a detailed evaluation and the extent of ischaemia must be defined in patients requiring revascularization. Evaluation includes a complete history, physical examination, laboratory profile, resting and exercise electrocardiography, chest X-ray and special studies including angiography.

Risk factors such as hypertension, diabetes, relevant family history, hypercholesterolaemia and smoking should be noted and wherever possible eliminated. Presence of other medical conditions which may have a bearing on management, such as, bleeding disorders, chronic obstructive airway disease, chronic steroid use, renal or liver failure, claudication and stroke should be explored.

Objective evidence of ischaemia must be sought and although a resting electrocardiogram (ECG) may provide valuable information regarding previous infarction, current ischaemia and arrhythmia, it may be normal in angina. Exercise ECG, carried out under carefully controlled conditions helps confirm the diagnosis and gives an objective measure of disability. Critical ischaemia at low work load indicates a poor natural history and a need for revascularization. Chest X-ray should be performed to determine the aortic and cardiac dimensions. As many patients are smokers pulmonary lesions may be detected.

Coronary angiography is performed to outline the coronary anatomy, define the extent of stenosis, the condition of the target vessels and estimate the left ventricular function.

Risk stratification

In the last decade several efforts have been made to identify significant preoperative risk factors which influence the outcome in patients undergoing coronary artery bypass graft (CABG). The identified risk factors are enumerated in *Table 2*. Preoperatively patients are stratified into various risk groups according to these risk factors. Parsonnet risk stratification is the most commonly adopted system in the UK (*Table 3*). A score is given for each risk factor and the total score obtained defines the risk, in per cent, for the individual patient.

Table 2. The most commonly identified risk factors in patients for CABG

Patient characteristics	Myocardial status	Perioperative conditions
Age	Priority of operation (urgent or emergency)	Perioperative myocardial infarction (MI)
Reoperation	Acute septal infarction	Accompanying valve disease
Renal dysfunction with high creatinine	Cardiogenic shock	Ventricular aneurysms
Peripheral vascular disease	Ejection fraction	Severity of coronary artery disease
Pulmonary dysfunction	Uncontrolled angina, NYHA, CHF	

Table 3. Parsonnet risk scores for various risk factors

Risk factor	Score	Risk factor	Score
1. Female gender	1	8. Reoperation	
		First reoperation	5
		Second reoperation	10
2. Morbid obesity (>1.5 of ideal weight)	3	9. Preoperative IABP	2
3. Diabetes (Unspecified)	3	10. Emergency surgery (Following PTCA or angiocatheter complication)	10
4. Hypertension (> 140 systolic)	3	11. Dialysis dependency (Peritoneal dialysis haemofiltration)	10
5. Age (years)		12. Catastrophic state	2–10
70–74	7	Actual structural defect	
75–79	12	Cardiogenic shock	
> 80	20	Acute renal failure	
6. Ejection fraction (%)		13. Rare circumstances	2–10
Good > 5	0	Paraplegia	
Fair 30–49	2	Pacemaker dependency	
Poor < 30	4	Congenital heart disease in adults Severe asthma	
		For valve surgery	
7. Left ventricular aneurysm	5	• Mitral valve	5
		PA pressures > 60 mmHg	8
		• Aortic valve	5
		Gradient >120 mmHg	7
		• Concomitant CABG	2

Each risk factor identified is given a score which is accumulated to give the risk in percentage for the individual patient.

Surgical revascularization

With the development of cardiopulmonary bypass and coronary angiography direct operation on the coronary arteries became possible and the first CABG was performed by Favorolo at the Cleveland Clinic in 1967. The long saphenous vein is the most commonly used conduit. There is, however, a significant occlusion rate of 10–15% at 1 year and thereafter a rate of 2–3%/year. There is ample evidence that use of arterial conduit improves the event-free survival in patients undergoing CABG. This is specifically so when the left internal mammary artery is grafted to the left anterior descending artery. For reasons yet to be determined the internal mammary artery is resistant to atherogenesis thus reliability, low occlusion rate and good long-term patency make it the conduit of choice.

Complications

1. Bleeding. Cardiopulmonary bypass damages the cellular and humoral components of blood. Platelets are reduced in number and may not function normally, while clotting factors may be reduced by as much as 50% and are major factors contributing to postoperative bleeding. Additional factors include pre-existing haematological problems, liver failure, renal failure, sepsis and allergic reactions to drugs or blood components. Continued bleeding and/or tamponade which occurs in 3% of patients requires urgent reoperation.

2. Perioperative myocardial infarction. Occurs in 4% of patients and although the diagnosis may be difficult it may manifest as low cardiac output. It is usually confirmed by persistent ECG changes, elevated cardiac enzymes and new regional wall motion on echocardiography.

3. Low cardiac output. Low cardiac output may result from tamponade, bleeding, inadequate pre-load, or poor myocardial function. Treatment entails treating the cause; bleeding should be investigated and treated, intracardiac filling optimized and rhythm disturbance treated. If the low output persists inotropic support is indicated.

If despite inotropic support low cardiac output persists haemodynamic support with intra-aortic balloon counterpulsion (IABP) may be required while the heart recovers. The IABP is inserted into the common femoral artery and threaded into the aorta until the tip lies just distal to the left subclavian artery. The balloon is triggered by the ECG to deflate in ventricular systole (thus reducing afterload) and inflate in diastole (displacing blood which perfuses the coronary arteries retrogradely). When the heart has recovered the balloon is removed. Complications include damage to the femoral artery, leg ischaemia and haemolysis.

4. Rhythm disturbances. Up to 30% of patients develop supraventricular dysarhythmias after cardiac surgery. These must be treated if they are persistent or cause haemodynamic compromise.

5. Infection. Adequate chest physiotherapy is the cornerstone of the prevention and treatment of postoperative pulmonary infections and basal collapse. Major wound infections are uncommon, occur in 1–2% of patients and may lead to sternal wound dehiscence and mediastinitis. The risk of serious wound infection is increased in the elderly, diabetics and patients undergoing bilateral internal mammary artery grafting.

Prognosis

Relief of symptoms and functional capacity are improved significantly following surgery when compared to medical treatment alone. Up to 90% of patients have complete relief of symptoms and require no further medication. In the remaining the symptoms are markedly reduced. It is important to note that surgery is not long lasting since any form of revascularization is not curative. Recurrence of symptoms is due to progressive disease in the native vessels and in the development of disease in the conduits. Hence, factors promoting atherogenesis must be carefully controlled, for example, hypercholesterolaemia should be aggressively managed, as should hypertension, smoking, diabetes and thyroid dysfunction. Many patients respond to medical treatment, but some will require revascularization. Surgical revascularization is associated with an increased operative mortality and is recommended only for patients with severe symptoms. Increasingly, coronary angioplasty (PRA) of new disease is utilized successfully.

Overall hospital mortality is 2–4%. An important indicator of performance, mortality is affected strongly by the preoperative risk factors of each individual patient as mentioned earlier. Hence, risk stratification, of which the Parsonnet scoring system is the most common, is used in cardiac surgery to predict outcome. Survival is also improved by the use of the internal mammary artery which has a superior long-term patency compared to other conduits.

Further reading

Metcalfe MJ, Lip GYH, Dargie HJ. Factors influencing continuing coronary artery bypass graft potency. *Cardiovascular Surgery,* 1994; **2:** 679–85.

Related topics of interest

Cardiovascular investigations – cardiac catheterization (p. 85)
Ischaemic heart disease – angina (p. 149)

CARDIAC TRANSPLANTATION

The first human heart transplant was performed by Christian Barnard in South Africa in 1967. Since then there have been substantial advances in this area, especially with immunosuppression and improved long-term outcome.

The introduction of effective immunosuppressive therapy, for example cyclosporin A in 1982, has led to greater results in such patients. Over 30 000 cardiac transplants have been performed world-wide and there are presently nine centres in the UK performing adult and/or paediatric heart transplantations.

Main indications

The main indication for adult cardiac transplantation is left ventricular failure, secondary to ischaemic heart disease or dilated cardiomyopathy. Other indications which are less common include cardiomyopathies, myocarditis and congenital heart disease.

Paediatric cardiac transplantation is usually for associated congenital heart disease or myocarditis.

Contraindication to cardiac transplantation

Absolute contraindications include other life-threatening illnesses (such as malignancy), hepatic failure, active infection, irreversible respiratory disease, increased pulmonary vascular resistance, diabetes mellitus with target organ damage, and current drug or alcohol abuse.

Relative contraindications include lack of social support, poor compliance, psychiatric illness, obesity, irreversible renal impairment and insulin-dependent diabetes.

The recipient

Recipient evaluation requires an assessment of whether the patient really does need a transplant, whether another treatment would be as effective, whether the patient desires to undergo transplantation, and whether there are any adverse features about the patient which would make the procedure inappropriate or too risky.

Patients who have been placed on a transplantation waiting list are reviewed regularly by their referring physician, but 19% of patients will die before being transplanted. The selection of the recipient is based upon ABO or blood compatibility, a heart which is of approximately matching size and the degree of urgency. If the recipient has a high pulmonary vascular resistance, the donor should be of the same weight or greater.

The donor

Organ transplantation in the UK is limited by the donor supply. Referrals are co-ordinated nationally by the United Kingdom Transplant Service.

Potential cardiac donors include patients who are less than 65 years, with no history of heart disease or cardiac surgery, normal 12 lead resting ECG, haemodynamically stable, and requiring only a low dosage of inotropes to maintain a reasonable cardiac output. Patients should fulfil criteria for brain death and have negative viral serology (HIV, hepatitis). Consent of next of kin should be available.

Patients are not suitable to be donors if there is a history of any malignancy, untreated infection, long periods of cardiac ischaemia, a history of disease or trauma involving the organs and long-standing diabetes, hypertension or cardiovascular disease.

Postoperative immunosuppression

This is based on a triple drug regime of cyclosporin A, azathioprine and prednisolone. Prednisolone is not used in children under five.

These drugs carry significant side-effects. For example, cyclosporin can result in hypertension and nephrotoxicity and requires regular monitoring by measurement of blood levels. Azathioprine can result in bone marrow toxicity, while steroids can cause Cushing's syndrome. Chronic immunosuppression can result in opportunistic bacterial, viral, protozoal and fungal infections and a theoretical risk of neoplasms.

Complications of cardiac transplantation

The main complications in patients following cardiac transplantation are organ rejection, infection and accelerated atherosclerosis in the donor heart.

Hyperacute rejection occurs when the recipient has pre-formed antibodies against the donor heart. Acute rejection is more common but there are few specific clinical signs of rejection. Regular cardiac biopsies are needed to asses this.

Accelerated graft atherosclerosis is a late complication which is characterized by occlusion of small cardiac vessels. It is diagnosed by angiography, autopsy or examination of the donor heart at re-transplantation. The risk factors for developing this problem are increased episodes of rejection, hypertension and smoking. It should be noted that since the transplanted heart is denervated, the problem of accelerated graft atherosclerosis usually presents as tachyarrhythmias, cardiac failure or sudden death.

Hypertension effects more than 75% of patients and is mainly due to cyclosporine therapy. Renal dysfunction is common in the early course, which may be due to cyclosporine nephrotoxicity. There is also an increased risk of malignancy in patients who are immunosuppressed.

The future

The size of the donor pool is the main limitation to cardiac transplantation. The future of cardiac replacement therapy includes new mechanical assist technologies, increasing the size of the donor pool (by raising public and professional awareness) and xenotransplantation. New, effective and safe methods of providing immunosuppression are needed.

Related topics of interest

CARDIAC TUMOURS

Cardiac tumours are rare with an incidence at *post mortem* of approximately 1:10 000. The majority of primary cardiac tumours are benign, with myxomas being the most common type (*Table 1*).

Metastatic tumours occur 20–40 times more frequently than primary cardiac tumours and are present in approximately 10% of patients with malignancy. The most common primary sites are lung and breast. Intracardiac involvement with Kaposi's sarcoma and lymphoma have been described in patients with AIDS.

Table 1. Primary cardiac tumours

Benign	Malignant
Myxoma	Rhabdomyosarcoma
Rhabdomyoma	Angiosarcoma
Fibroma	Fibrosarcoma
Lipoma	
Haemangioma	
Papillary fibroelastoma	

Primary cardiac tumours

1. Myxoma. This tumour can occur in any chamber, although it is found most commonly in the left atrium (75%) arising from the inter-atrial septum in the region of the fossa ovalis. It is typically a solitary gelatinous pedunculated mass, which prolapses through the mitral or tricuspid valve. The size is variable and the tumour may fill the left atrium. It is thought to be of endothelial or endocardial origin and fragments of the tumour frequently lead to systemic emboli. Multiple tumours occur rarely and there is a rare familial form associated with pigmented skin lesions and peripheral or endocrine neoplasms.

(a) Symptoms:
- Constitutional, including lethargy, myalgia, fever, weight loss and syncope.
- Dyspnoea, gradual onset exertional dyspnoea or acute severe pulmonary oedema.
- Embolic, these may involve any organ resulting in fits, hemiplegia, acute limb ischaemia or myocardial infarction.

(b) Clinical features: a low grade fever may be present. The most important physical signs are a loud first heart sound, a mid-diastolic murmur and an early diastolic tumour 'plop' (as the pedunculated tumour comes to an abrupt halt). Right atrial myxomas may produce signs of right ventricular dysfunction or pulmonary infarction.

(c) Investigations: the ESR is frequently raised. Chest X-ray may show enlargement of the left atrial appendage and possibly pulmonary oedema. Transthoracic echocardiography allows characterization of the tumour by assessing its size, location, points of attachment, mobility and consistency. Transoesophageal echocardiography may provide more detailed information.

(d) Treatment: surgical removal is successful in the majority of patients. Occasionally atrial septectomy and an inter-atrial patch is necessary. Recurrence of the myxoma is rare, although follow up for the first 5 years is recommended.

2. *Rhabdomyoma.* Rhabdomyomas are the most common cardiac tumours of childhood. About 85% are seen in children below the age of 15 years and the majority of these affect children below 1 year. They are thought to be hamartomas and occur with equal frequency between the left and right ventricles. Rhabdomyomas are frequently multiple and there is a strong association with tuberose sclerosis. These tumours are variable in size and may obstruct the ventricular cavities soon after birth or later in childhood. They may also interfere with cardiac conduction. If the tumour is single and obstructive, then surgical excision is the treatment of choice.

3. *Fibroma.* These are the second most common form of cardiac tumour in children. They are typically solitary, solid, echogenic mass lesions and are located in the left ventricular free wall or interventricular septum. Tumours involving the interventricular septum may give the appearance of

asymmetrical septal hypertrophy and should not be confused with HOCM. Echocardiography will demonstrate the tumour and screen patients for regrowth following surgery. Cardiac surgery may be problematic and it is often difficult to secure complete removal of the tumour.

4. Other benign tumours. Lipomas, papillary fibroelastomas and haemangiomas are rarely seen in the heart. Intra-cardiac lipomas are true benign neoplasms and normally appear as small lobulated sub-endocardial masses at *post mortem*. Myocardial or endocardial lipomas may interfere with cardiac conduction or obstruct intracardiac blood flow. Papillary fibroelastomas usually arise from the mitral and aortic valves or endocardium. Emboli and valvular dysfunction are rare complications. Haemangiomas occur at any age and in any part of the heart. They occur in the atrio-ventricular node and interventricular septum, resulting in heart block and sudden death. Endocrine-secreting tumours such as pheochromocytoma are also rarely seen.

Primary malignant tumours

The majority of primary malignant cardiac tumours are sarcomas and are usually associated with a poor prognosis. Angiosarcoma is the most common malignant tumour and most commonly involves the right side of the heart or the pericardium. These tumours frequently involve the vena cava, tricuspid valve and involvement of the pericardium leads to clinical signs of pericardial effusion or tamponade.

Echocardiography may demonstrate the tumour and an associated pericardial effusion.

Metastases are often present at diagnosis and the prognosis is poor.

CARDIOMYOPATHY

Cardiomyopathies are defined as a group of diseases involving the heart muscle where the aetiology is unknown. They are, therefore, not secondary to valvular, congenital, hypertensive, pericardial or ischaemic heart disease. Since the term was defined, some predisposing conditions have been recognized. The term 'secondary cardiomyopathy' is, therefore, applied to myocardial diseases where the cause is known, whilst idiopathic cardiomyopathy refers to diseases of heart muscle of unknown cause or associations. Secondary cardiomyopathy may be:

- Inflammatory – Post viral (Coxsackie, ECHO viruses, etc.), bacterial, toxoplasmosis, rickettsial, spirochaetal, parasitic (Chagas disease), vasculitic (Kawasaki's disease)
- Endocrine/metabolic – Acromegaly, thyrotoxicosis, myxoedema, uraemia, thiamine deficiency, phaeochromocytoma
- Toxic – Cobalt, alcohol, bleomycin, adriamycin, corticosteroids, tricyclic antidepressants
- Infiltrative – Amyloidosis, haemochromatosis, sarcoidosis, leukaemia
- Neuromuscular – Duchenne muscular dystrophy, Friedreich's ataxia, myotonia dystrophica
- Miscellaneous – Peripartum cardiomyopathy, collagen disorder, drug hypersensitivity

Primary cardiomyopathy

Types

- Dilated.
- Hypertrophic.
- Restrictive.

Dilated cardiomyopathy (DCM)

This is characterized by impaired systolic function of the ventricles and chamber dilatation causing congestive heart failure. The incidence is 5–8 per 100 000 population per year. It is three times more common in the Afro-Caribbean population as compared to Caucasian. Twenty per cent have a first degree relative with the condition. Autosomal inheritance patterns are often found, some have autosomal recessive and sex-linked inheritance. Angiotensin converting enzyme DD genotype has been described.

Histopathological examination demonstrates variation in myocyte size, and some cells are hypertrophied, others atrophic with interstitial fibrosis, cellular infiltration and myocardial degeneration.

Dilatation of all four chambers and wall thinness is characteristic on echocardiography. Valves and coronary arteries are otherwise normal, although ventricular dilatation may lead to mitral and tricuspid incompetence. Thrombus may be found in the dilated chambers.

A similar picture is seen in alcohol and thyrotoxicosis related: it is speculated that a viral myocarditis (primarily Coxsackie) may initiate an autoimmune process culminating in the final picture of DCM. However, less than 15% of patients with myocarditis progress to cardiomyopathy and less than 10% of patients with cardiomyopathy have evidence of myocarditis on biopsy (polymorphonuclear leucocytosis and other inflammatory cell infilteration with interstitial fibrosis).

Symptoms and signs. Congestive cardiac failure (CCF) and stroke / thromboembolism (which occur in 15–20%) are common, although in some patients the presenting symptom is angina in the absence of coronary artery disease. Onset of symptoms of CCF is usually gradual but may be acute following an influenzal-type illness when myocarditis is suspected. There is usually evidence of cardiomegaly, often with a third heart sound and evidence of mitral and tricuspid regurgitation, due to myocardial dilatation.

Investigations. These should exclude secondary causes – alcoholism, thyroid function, iron studies, etc. Abnormal liver function tests and a raised MCV may be due to high alcohol intake.

Chest x-ray to assess chamber dilatation, interstitial oedema and pleural effusions.

ECG, though non-diagnostic, is usually abnormal and may show sinus tachycardia, ventricular arrhythmias, atrial fibrillation, bundle branch block or non-specific repolarization changes without Q waves.

Echocardiogram shows dilated left ventricle with poor contraction and usually ejection fraction of less than 35%. The right ventricle may show similar changes.

Prognosis. About 20% of patients die within 1 year. Patients with persisting signs of congestive heart failure, despite full treatment, ejection fraction of less than 25%, ventricular arrhythmias and Afro-Caribbeans have a particularly poor prognosis. Patients with higher ejection fraction, with completely controlled cardiac failure and reasonable exercise capacity, have a better outlook and can survive up to 10 years or longer.

In the minority of patients, the heart size and cardiac function improves considerably and there may be a sub-group who had myocarditis (healed) or alcoholic cardiomyopathy.

Treatment. This is treatment for heart failure, and includes diuretics and ACE inhibitors. Digoxin is helpful in controlling atrial fibrillation and reduces need for hospital admissions, although it does not prolong life (the DIG study). There is some evidence that beta blockers, such as metoprolol can improve quality of life and morbidity, but not mortality in idiopathic DCM. Carvediolol is a beta blocker with vasodilator properties which has been shown to have beneficial effects. The value of calcium antagonists is uncertain, although the PRAISE study has suggested that the long-acting dihydropyridine calcium antagonist, amlodipine, may have a survival advantage in non-ischaemic DCM. Transplantation is an option for suitable patients.

Antithrombotic therapy is necessary, and warfarin is indicated in atrial arrhythmias, severely impaired cardiac function and the presence of thrombus.

Hypertrophic cardiomyopathy (HCM)

The hallmark is unexplained hypertrophy which typically involves the interventricular septum (asymmetric hypertrophy) or other parts of the ventricles. For example, the interventricular septum being thicker than the posterior wall (ratio > 1.3:1). In 85% there is gradient across the outflow tract of the left ventricle, often termed subaortic stenosis. In some cases, there is no resting gradient but this can be provoked by exercise, isoprenaline, nitrates and Valsalva manoeuvre. In 15% there is no gradient.

Genetics and prevalence
Incidence – 0.2%
Autosomal dominant with high degree of penetrance
Equal sex distribution

Histology
Hypertrophy of muscle and disorganization (Whorled pattern)
Disorganization of myofibritis
Cellular disarray
Fibrosis

Presentation and symptoms
Occurs in infants, children, adults, elderly
May be asymptomatic
Syncope
Angina
Breathlessness
Palpitations
Sudden death related to malignant arrhythmias

The marked hypertrophy and consequent increase in oxygen demand gives rise to angina, in the presence of normal coronary arteries. The hypertrophied muscle is stiff, causing left atrial enlargement and pulmonary venous hypertension, leading to dyspnoea. The hypertrophied septum narrows the outflow tract and in combination with a small left ventricular cavity and dynamic contraction may lead to a venturi effect which sucks in the anterior mitral valve leaflet giving rise to a dynamic outflow tract obstruction especially under conditions of increased sympathetic tone (for example, exercise, isoprenaline infusion or during phase II of the Valsalva manoeuvre), or reduced left ventricular volume (for example, amyl nitrate inhalation, upright position, dehydration), leading to syncope.

Disturbed function of the anterior mitral leaflet may also explain the mitral incompetence. Arrhythmias are a common problem, especially ventricular tachyarrhythmias (which may lead to sudden death) and atrial fibrillation (which is often poorly tolerated due to loss of atrial contribution to left ventricular filling).

Signs. Typical physical signs include left ventricular hypertrophy, with a forceful apex beat, and a systolic murmur of LV outflow tract obstruction or mitral incompetence, and a loud fourth heart sound. The apex beat often has a double impulse due to enhanced atrial systole, due to hypertrophied stiff ventricle. If there is evidence of obstruction the pulse is typically small in volume and has a jerky ill-sustained upstroke. In severe cases, with right ventricular involvement, prominent 'a' waves in JVP are seen.

ECG and CXR. In the majority (90%) the ECG is abnormal but not diagnostic. The ECG may show evidence of left ventricular hypertrophy with strain. Abnormal Q wave or evidence of subendocardial ischaemia with deep T-wave inversion in precordial leads are occasionally present. The latter is often seen in apical HCM (described in Japan) where the left ventricle is spade-like with gradient within the left ventricle. Prognosis in this type is favourable. In 20% there is a Wolff–Parkinson–White type tracing.

The chest x-ray is non-diagnostic and is usually normal in the initial stages, but later cardiac enlargement with prominent left atrium is present.

On echocardiography there is LV hypertrophy, premature aortic valve closure and systolic anterior motion of the anterior mitral valve leaflet; the latter correlates closely with presence of outflow tract obstruction.

Cardiac catheterization. High left ventricular end-diastolic pressure. Subaortic pressure gradient in

HOCM is provoked by exercise, isoprenaline, Valsalva manoeuvre. Mild elevation of pulmonary artery and wedge pressure with prominent 'a' waves. There may be gradient between apex and body of left ventricle. Left ventricular angiogram shows a hypertrophied left ventricle, with 50% showing mitral incompetence. The left ventricular cavity is small with vigorous contraction. Coronary arteries in the majority are normal.

Prognosis and natural history. Patients' symptoms may remain mild and stable in many adults for years. In children, prognosis is poor and annual mortality is around 5% (in adults it is around 2–3%). Cardiac dilatation, syncope, atrial fibrillation, clinical evidence or Holter evidence of ventricular tachycardia and sudden death in patients or siblings are bad prognostic signals. Sudden death occurs when previous 24 h ECG had shown ventricular tachycardia. Another adverse feature is an abnormal blood pressure response to exercise, with a fall or failure to rise more than 20 mm Hg. In very late stages in some survivors there is cardiomegaly, suggesting poor prognosis. The mode of death is usually malignant arrhythmia or acute haemodynamic disturbance.

The condition is often familial and adolescents with a 'malignant' family history (for example, one or two primary relatives with sudden death before age 45 years) are at increased risk of death.

Treatment. The aims of management are the treatment of symptoms, and the prevention of sudden death.

Angina. Beta blocker, may also reduce gradient. Avoid nitrates in HOCM (may increase gradient). Calcium antagonists with negative chronotropic effects (such as verapamil or diltiazem) may also improve relaxation of ventricles.

Sudden death. Beta blockers have not been proven to be effective, although commonly prescribed for this condition. There is some favourable observational evidence with Amiodarone. Automative defibrillators in high risk patients with frequent syncope/VT.

Surgical treatment. Excision of interventricular septum to reduce gradient, combined with mitral valve replacement for mitral regurgitation. These procedures are not widely used. Recently dual chamber pacemakers programmed with a short A-V delay to pre-excite the ventricle have been shown to reduce gradient and improve exercise tolerance Recent reports of successful reduction in septal hypertrophy and reduction in LV outflow tract gradient by selectively occluding the 1st septal branch of the left anterior descending artery still remain controversial and unproven.

Restrictive cardiomyopathy This may be due to infiltrative disease or idiopathic. The condition is rare. Possible identifiable causes include sarcoidosis, scleroderma, radiation, amyloid disease or haemochromatosis. Less understood is Loffler's endocarditis due to marked eosinophilia.

The main abnormality is restriction of ventricular relaxation due to rigid wall. Systolic function is preserved.

Symptoms, signs and haemodynamics. The common symptoms are shortness of breath and signs of congestive cardiac failure. The atria are dilated, as seen on echocardiogram, without dilation of ventricles. Left and right ventricular end-diastolic pressures are near-normal, although, in the majority, it is 5 mm more in the left ventricle than in the right. The clinical picture in constrictive pericarditis is similar, however, in the latter, the end-diastolic pressures are mostly equal. In both conditions there is rapid decrease in diastolic pressure with rapid rise in early diastole and plateau (there may be a square root sign). In atrial trace there is rapid y descent and it is difficult to differentiate this condition from constrictive pericarditis. Myocardial biopsy, CT scanning and MRI, to assess pericardial thickening, and chest x-ray, to show calcification, may be helpful. Constriction of pericardium after cardiac surgery presents a similar picture and is a difficult diagnostic problem.

Investigations and management. In Loffler's syndrome there is eosinophilia >1500/mm^3. In Churg–Strauss syndrome there is also asthma, nasal polyposis and necrotizing vasculitis. Besides evidence of cardiac failure, thromboembolism is common.

Myocardial biopsy shows inflammatory eosinophilia, myocarditis, fibrosis and areas of thrombosis.

ECG is non-diagnostic and can include non-specific T-wave changes, arrhythmias, atrial fibrillation and conduction defects.

- Echocardiogram. Atrial dilatation and obliteration of apex by thrombosis.
- Haemodynamics. Same as other restrictive conditions.

Treatment is often difficult and aimed at improving cardiac failure. Digoxin in amyloid disease may bind with amyloid cardiac tissue and should be given with caution. Treatment is aimed at treating CHF. Steroids/cytotoxic drugs have been tried with variable results.

Endomyocardial fibrosis (EMF)

Occurs in tropical countries and other parts of Africa. There is extensive fibrosis of myocardium and endocardium involving mitral and tricuspid valves. The signs and symptoms are those of severe cardiac failure with poor prognosis. Thromboembolism is common.

Further reading

Oakley C. Aetiology, diagnosis, investigation and management of the cardiomyopathies. *British Medical Journal,* 1997; **315**: 1520–24.

CARDIOVASCULAR INVESTIGATIONS – CARDIAC CATHETERIZATION

Cardiac catheterization enables anatomical and physiological assessment of cardiac lesions. In many situations it also provides the option for a therapeutic modality which is less invasive than surgery. It has come a long way since the German radiologist Werner Forssman negotiated a ureteric catheter into his own heart and walked to the radiology department for a confirmatory x-ray, whilst looking for means to rapidly deliver drugs into the heart.

Intubation of cardiac chambers allows:

- Accurate pressure measurements in individual cardiac chambers which can be correlated to different phases of the cardiac cycle using the ECG.
- Sampling of blood for oximetry which allows accurate detection and quantitation of intracardiac shunts.
- Injection of radiological contrast media allowing accurate study of cardiac chambers and vasculature (angiography).
- Measurement of cardiac output using dye and thermodilution techniques.
- Therapeutic procedures on arteries, valves and congenital defects.

Pressure measurements

Right heart catheterization is carried out from the femoral, antecubital and sometimes (in ITU settings) the subclavian and internal jugular veins. Pressures are measured from the right atrium, ventricle, pulmonary artery and pulmonary capillary wedge positions.

The right atrial pressure wave has positive a, c and v waves produced by atrial systole, tricuspid valve closure (initial ventricular systole) and venous filling respectively. Negative x descent is produced by the tricuspid ring descent during ventricular ejection. The y descent is due to tricuspid valve opening, allowing atrial pressure to rapidly fall and equalize to ventricular diastolic.

V waves are prominent in tricuspid regurgitation. In constrictive pericarditis, where the jugular venous pressure is elevated, the y descent is quite prominent because of rapid initial filling of the right ventricle until sudden restriction to ventricular filling occurs (corresponding to the pericardial knock). In contrast, cardiac tamponade does not permit initial rapid ventricular filling and the y descent is obliterated.

The mean right atrial pressure is 0–6 mmHg. Higher pressures are seen in congestive heart failure or raised ventricular wall stiffness when pulmonary hypertension or stenosis is present.

Right ventricular systolic pressure up to 30 mmHg is considered normal. Diastolic pressure is approximately equal to the atrial pressure (a wave) when the tricuspid valve is open. Systolic pressure is elevated in pulmonary stenosis and hypertension. In pulmonary stenosis a pressure drop occurs across the pulmonary valve with systolic pulmonary arterial pressure often below 15 mmHg.

Normal pulmonary arterial pressures are below 30 mmHg systolic and 18 mmHg mean. High PA pressures are found in pulmonary thrombo-embolism, primary pulmonary hypertension and left heart disease. The conditions are differentiated by the capillary wedge pressure: in left heart disease the pulmonary wedge pressure is high but it is normal in pulmonary thromboembolism and primary pulmonary hypertension.

Pulmonary capillary wedge pressure approximates left atrial pressure. By wedging the measuring catheter into pulmonary arterioles forward blood flow stops and arteriolar pressures fall to venular and thus left atrial pressures – the pressure trace records back pressure from the pulmonary veins which approximately equals left atrial pressure. Wedge pressure waveforms are somewhat similar to right atrial with a, c and v waves and x and y descents. The a wave is prominent in mitral stenosis (where the patient is still in sinus rhythm). A prominent v wave is seen in mitral regurgitation.

Left heart catheterization is usually carried out using a percutaneous Seldinger technique entry into the femoral artery. Using a cannulating needle a guidewire is fed into the femoral artrery over which a catheter can be threaded under fluoroscopic control into the aorta or left ventricle. Sometimes direct cut-down to the brachial artery is employed, especially where there is peripheral vascular disease.

Systolic and diastolic aortic pressure is the same as peripheral arterial pressure and is raised in hypertension. LV systolic pressure exceeds aortic by more than 10 mmHg in aortic valve stenosis. The end diastolic pressure is raised in the left ventricle in left ventricular failure or as a result of hypertrophy, e.g. hypertension, hypertrophic cardiomyopathy or aortic stenosis. In infiltrative disease diastolic pressures can be high.

Transatrial septal puncture allows left heart catheterization from the venous system and is sometimes used when a mechanical aortic valvular prosthesis makes retrograde LV entry impractical. It also affords balloon mitral valvuloplasty in mitral stenosis.

Saturations

Intracardiac oxygen saturation can assess shunts. Right-sided oxygen saturations are usually between 60 and 80%: the venous blood returning via the superior vena cava is relatively desaturated whereas that from the inferior vena cava is less so as the kidney has a high blood flow but low oxygen uptake. Venous admixture occurs in the right atrium.

Left-sided saturations are usually over 96% (lower in heart failure and pulmonary disease). In left to right shunts there is a rise in saturation at the level of the shunt and beyond. For example, in an ASD there is a step-up in oxygen saturation in the right atrium as compared to systemic venous saturation and in a VSD step-up occurs at the right ventricular and pulmonary artery level. In right to left shunts, in congenital cyanotic heart disease, a drop in saturation occurs at the level of the shunt.

Angiography

Injection into the left ventricle allows assessment of its overall and segmental contractility and allows assessment of any mitral regurgitation. The normal LV EF is around 70%. Aortic root injections allow estimates of severity of aortic incompetence.

Angiography remains the only widely available and reliable anatomical assessment of the coronary arteries. By selective cannulation of coronary ostia, using special pre-shaped catheters, it is possible to study coronary artery filling and correlate this information to exercise ECG, left ventricular wall motion and perfusion defects noted on radionuclide scanning.

Special procedures

Swan–Ganz catheterization. A balloon-tipped catheter introduced into a central vein, e.g. internal jugular, passes through the right heart chambers into the pulmonary artery, the inflated balloon helping it to float passively. It is often used in ITU monitoring as it can be advanced without fluoroscopic control. Measurement of right-sided and pulmonary wedge pressures is helpful in guiding management in situations like cardiogenic shock and right ventricular infarction.

Therapeutic procedures. Percutaneous transluminal coronary angioplasty (PTCA), stenting and related procedures. Using special guiding systems it is possible to steer a guidewire across coronary stenoses and place a miniature balloon-tipped catheter astride the narrowing. Using several atmospheres of pressure it is possible to stretch these lesions. The result – a mixture of plaque compression, intimal disruption and sometimes (hopefully localized) dissection – usually leads to an improvement of coronary blood flow into the stenosed artery and affords symptomatic relief. Complications of the procedure naturally include more widespread vessel disruption or closure requiring urgent bypass surgery or stent (stainless steel mesh) placement. In addition, there is overall a 30–50% chance of restenosis occurring at the site of PTCA. There is some evidence that elective stenting reduces chances of restenosis.

Similar procedures involve using high-speed diamond-dusted burrs (rotablators) to fragment atheromata or using atheroma shaving (atherectomy)/extracting (TEC) devices to de-bulk coronary lesions as an adjunct to PTCA.

Valvuloplasty. It is possible to position balloon-tipped catheters across stenosed pulmonary, mitral (trans-septally or retrogradely through the left ventricle) and aortic valves. These high tensile balloons can be inflated to several atmospheres, stretching the stenosed valve, ideally leading to commissural separation with minimal post-procedural valve incompetence. Balloon dilatation is also used in coarctation of aorta.

Closure of congenital defects (atrial septal defects and patent ductus arteriosus, rarely ventricular septal defects). It is sometimes possible to place special umbrella-like devices across congenital defects enabling closure using special delivery systems. These procedures would ordinarily have required cardiac surgery. Transcatheter closure represents an important advance in the management of some congenital heart diseases.

Transposition of the great arteries is an important neonatal emergency associated with significant de-oxygenation and cardiac failure. It is possible to provide some relief to these infants by creating an atrial septal defect by a trans-septal balloon catheter introduced through femoral umbilical vein. The resulting admixture of blood allows these very sick infants to be taken up for corrective surgery.

Further reading

Norrell M, de Belder M, Mills P, de Feyter P (eds). Interventional cardiology. *Heart*, October 1997; **78** (Supplement 2).

CARDIOVASCULAR INVESTIGATIONS – ECHOCARDIOGRAPHY

Echocardiography is a widely used, safe investigation for patients with suspected cardiac disease. Ultrasonic waves are directed from a transducer towards the heart, and pictures generated by the reflection of the ultrasonic waves (echos) from tissue interfaces. The pictures are constructed by combining information about the strength of the echos and the time delay between emission of the ultrasonic waves and return of the echos. Echocardiography is most frequently performed from outside the thorax, either through the rib spaces or from the subcostal approach. Trans-oesophageal echocardiography (TOE) is performed from the oesophagus, with the probe mounted on the end of an endoscope.This provides high resolution and higher quality images since the probe is closer to the heart, and intervening ribs are not present. Recently available is intravasular ultrasound (IVUS), where the probe is mounted on a catheter which can be passed down coronary arteries. This imaging method is finding application from imaging deployment of intracoronary stents. The three main imaging modalities used in the assessment of cardiac structure and function are summarized as follows:

M-Mode

Historically this was the first type of echocardiography. A one dimensional image of the heart is displayed. The frame rate (no. of pictures/sec) is greater than 2-dimensional echocardiography, which therefore improves temporal resolution. M-mode is useful in assessing the dynamics of cardaic motion. Superimposition of colour Doppler (colour M-mode) allows accurate timing of blood flow through cardiac chambers and valves.

2-dimensional imaging

Emission of a fan of ultrasonic waves enables a 2-dimensional image (slice) to be generated. This can provide more detail on morphological structure of the heart than M-mode. Images are commonly recorded from the apical, parasternal and subcostal regions (orthogonal planes) to enable the observer to formulate a complete picture about cardiac morphology.

Doppler

Doppler echocardiography enables evaluation of the direction and velocity of blood flow (and myocardial motion) through the cardiac chambers and blood vessels. The Doppler effect relies upon the change in frequency of the ultrasonic wave when it encounters a moving object. The frequency of shift is related to direction and velocity of motion. Continuous-wave Doppler detects blood flow at any point along the ultrasonic beam, such that there is no spatial resolution along the beam, and that the envelope of velocities is likely to be very broad. Pulsed-wave Doppler permits sampling from a certain preselected 'sample volume' within the heart. This enables greater spatial accuracy. Unfortunately pulsed-wave Doppler has problems with the detection of high frequency jets (such as aortic stenosis or mitral regurgitation), which are better quantified with continuous wave Doppler. Colour Doppler makes recordings of Doppler frequency shifts over on arc (much like 2-dimensional echocardiography), and constructs a colour map of flow towards and away from the transducer which is superimposed on the 2-dimensional image. This simplifies detection of abnormal blood flow through the heart and great vessels, although pulsed- and continuous-wave Doppler is still required for quantificative assessment.

Clinical applications

Myocardial disease. Echocardiography permits accurate assessment of chamber size, wall thickness, and contractile function. Global abnormalities in left ventricular function can be reliably differentiated from regional wall motion abnormalities, such as those found in coronary artery disease. Left ventricular hypertrophy can be accurately identified and quantitatively measured. Exercise stress echocardiography is an extension of this technique now being used for the detection of regional wall motion abnormalities in coronary artery disease. TOE is finding application for monitoring of cardiac contractilty during high risk surgical proceedures.

Valvular disease. M-mode and 2-dimensional echocardiography are of particular value for detecting structural valvular abnormalities and associated chamber dilatation or hypertrophy.

Doppler echocardiography provides important information on the presence and severity of valvular lesions. Medium to large vegetations can be identified using transthoracic echocardiography in patients with infective endocarditis. TOE is particularly useful for assessment of prosthetic heart valves, and detecting vegetations in infective endocarditis.

Great vessel disease. TOE is now the principal investigation for aortic disease, such as dissection and aneurysm, because of the close proximity of the probe to the aorta.

Congenital heart disease. Echocardiography has transformed investigation of congenital heart disease, since the relationships of the venous supply, atria, ventricles, and great vessels can be readily determined. TOE is being used to assess which septal defects are amenable to trans-catheter device closure.

Other applications. Echocardiography is the most accuate technique available for detection of pericardial effusions. Intracardiac tumours (including thrombi) are well seen with echocardiography. TOE has found application in the detection of left atrial thrombi.

CARDIOVASCULAR INVESTIGATIONS – RADIONUCLIDE INVESTIGATIONS

A number of radiopharmaceuticals are available to investigate different aspects of cardiac function. The most popular and well-known is myocardial perfusion scan. The other radionuclide tests look at viability of ischaemic myocardium, ejection fraction, wall motion abnormalities, infarction, and myocardial metabolism.

Myocardial perfusion studies

Radiopharmaceuticals. Thallium-201 (^{201}Tl). Thallium-201 is a well established myocardial perfusion agent which is widely used. Following injection it immediately distributes in the myocardium according to myocardial perfusion – in areas of previous myocardial infarction, no redistribution occurs, allowing distinction between normal, ischaemic and infarcted myocardium. The mechanism of uptake is similar to potassium. The initial uptake of thallium peaks at 10 minutes, then it redistributes (washout plasma $t_{1/2}$ of 1 h). Usually, the injection is given intravenously at peak exercise and images obtained immediately following exercise (to detect ischaemia) and rest images 4 h later to allow for redistribution.

Further elucidation of myocardial function may allow detection of hibernating or stunned myocardium, thallium is reinjected at rest followed by early and late (up to 24 h) images. Thallium is the agent of choice for detection of hibernating myocardium – the latter shows up as very late redistribution. The evidence suggests that revascularization of such areas predicts return of myocardial contractility.

The relative disadvantage of thallium compared to Technetium agents is its higher radiation dose to the patient and relatively poorer images, due to high uptake by liver, lung and skeletal muscle.

Technetium (^{99}Tc^m) based myocardial perfusion agents. The Technetium based agents include ^{99}Tc^m Tetrofosmin, ^{99}Tc^m SestaMIBI (MIBI), and ^{99}Tc^m Teboroxime. Higher gamma ray energy (140 keV) and shorter half-life (6.2 h) of ^{99}Tc^m results in less radiation to the patient (typical study EDE = 7 mSv) and sharper images in particular of the posterior and inferior walls. These agents fix in the myocardium proportional to perfusion with no significant washout and redistribution. Two injections (one at rest, and one at exercise) are required. Both 1 day and 2 day protocols are used with satisfactory results. The additional advantages of Technetium based agents are better resolution, faster images and that the imaging need not immediately follow exercise, however gastrointestinal excretion may cause image reconstruction problems.

Technetium Teboroxime with fast washout time (7 minutes), is only suitable for departments with multi-headed cameras capable of fast imaging (less than 10 minutes). It is most suitable for repeat quick studies on the same patient.

Myocardial perfusion studies have a sensitivity of 85%, specificity 73% and accuracy of 80% for diagnosing ischaemic heart disease.

Indications for myocardial perfusion studies

- Patient with angina and right or left bundle branch block.
- Patient with physical disability, unable to perform exercise tolerance test (ETT).
- Sub-maximal ETT due to shortness of breath, tiredness, etc.
- Inconclusive ET.
- To further evaluate ET: symptoms discrepant with the result.
- Estimate the size and location of fixed (infarcted) and reversible ischaemic area of the myocardium.
- To evaluate the significance of a known coronary artery stenosis.

'Stress' test for myocardial perfusion studies

The choice of 'stress' depends on the physicians preference, hospital set up and patient condition. Vasodilators are only suitable for myocardial perfusion and are not used to detect ECG changes or myocardial motion abnormalities.

Physical exercise. Graded exercise using treadmill or bicycle.

Pharmacological 'stress'

- Dobutamine. This is a beta-adrenergic agent with ionotropic and chronotropic effect on the heart. It is used in patients unable to exercise. The infusion rate is increased until symptoms, ECG changes or maximum heart rate are achieved.
- Arbutamine. Similar to dobutamine, however with more predictable chronotropic effects: The heart rate is gradually increased until end point criteria are reached.
- Adenosine. This agent is a potent vasodilator increasing myocardial perfusion by up to six times (in physical exercise there is usually a three- to four-fold increase in myocardial blood flow). Adenosine is infused at a dose of 0.84 mg/kg over a period of 7 minutes and the radiopharmaceutical is injected at 3 minutes. It has a short half life of 30 sec. Minor side-effects are common (up to 60% of patients) and include shortness of breath, headache, chest and neck pain, however major side-effects (arrythmias and AV block) are rare and should be watched for. It is contraindicated in patients with asthma as it is also a bronchoconstrictor.
- Dipyridamole. Inhibits the breakdown of endogenously produced adenosine in the body. Its affects are similar to adenosine, however as the block is prolonged the side-effects last longer.
- Combination of vasodilators and exercise. Some centres combine low level exercise (40 W) with adenosine infusion.

Twelve-lead ECG monitoring is essential when using treadmill, bicycle, dobutamine or arbutamine to assess ST-T changes. When using adenosine or dipyridamole a three-lead monitor is usually sufficient to detect arrythmias.

Multigated ventriculography (MUGA)

The most common method of performing the test is to label the red cells with $^{99}Tc^m$ and acquire 16 or 32 frames per heart beat by synchronizing ('gating') imaging with ECG. The ejection fraction, systolic filling rate, diastolic emptying rate, and wall motion abnormalities can then be calculated. The response of the heart to stress/exercise is assessed by measuring the changes in cardiac parameters. The normal global left ventricular ejection fraction using this method is >40%. The test is operator independent and gives consistent results. EF estimates do not depend upon assumptions about the heart's shape (in contrast to contrast ventriculograpyy and echocardiography) and are ideal for serial reassessment of EF.

Infarct imaging

Several agents have been used to assess the presence and extent of an infarct. The best known of these agents is $^{99}Tc^m$-labelled pyrophosphate, which is taken up by the infarcted myocardium. Best imaging time is 48–72 h after the infarct. It has a sensitivity of up to 95% and specificity of 80%. Other agents such as radiolabelled myosin antibodies have also been used. It is possible to assess the infarcted myocardium using myocardial perfusion studies (negative scan). These tests are rarely carried out in UK except for research purposes.

Positron emission tomography (PET)

In PET scanning, unlike the standard nuclear medicine scan where a gamma emitting radionuclide is used, a positron emitting radionuclide is used. Immediately after a positron (positively charged electron, e^+) is released from the nucleus it interacts with neighbouring electrons (e^-) and is entirely converted to energy (matter–antimatter interaction) thus emitting two high energy (511 keV) gamma rays in opposite directions. It is possible to detect these opposing coincidental gamma rays and locate the site of the interaction. With this technique it is possible to directly observe and quantify the distribution of agents such as nitrogen (^{13}N ammonia), oxygen (^{15}O-water), ^{18}F glucose (fluorine-^{18}FDG). Using these agents it is possible to image the viable myocardium independent of the state of perfusion. This technique requires a PET camera and a cyclotron to produce positron emitting radionuclides, which are at present expensive and only available in larger centres. In future standard two-headed gamma cameras may be able to image these agents satisfactorily.

Other cardiac nuclear medicine imaging tests
- ^{123}I MIBG accumulates at the adrenergic receptor sites and has been used to map the adrenergic receptor sites of myocardium.
- ^{123}I MIBG accumulates at the adrenergic receptor sites and has been used to map the adrenergic receptor sites of myocardium.
- Labelled fatty acids have been used to image myocardial metabolism.

Further reading

Zaret BL, Wackers FJ. Nuclear cardiology. Review article I. *New England Journal of Medicine,* 1993; **329:** 775–83.

Zaret BL, Wackers FJ. Nuclear cardiology. Review article II. *New England Journal of Medicine,* 1993; **329:** 855–63.

CARDIOVASCULAR INVESTIGATIONS – THE ELECTROCARDIOGRAPH AND EXERCISE STRESS TESTING

Exercise testing

The patient exercises at increasing levels of exercise until a predetermined point (e.g target heart rate greater than 160 beats per minute) or until exhaustion or other limiting symptoms, such as chest pain or dyspnoea. Treadmill exercise is favoured in the U.K. (e.g. Bruce protocol), whereas in other countries bicycle testing is prefered.

The following variables are documented:

- Total exercise time and total workload (an indirect measure of oxygen uptake).
- Symptoms during the test.
- Heart rate and blood pressure.
- Arrhythmias documented.
- ST and T wave changes on the ECG.

The classic ischaemic response is of 'planar ST depression' occuring during exercise (equal to more than 2 mm flat or downsloping) with resolution during rest. However, the ECG may be altered by many factors other than ischaemia, so that the ECG response is not specific. Important confounders are drugs (e.g. Digoxin), electrolyte abnormalities (hypokalaemia), changes in sympathetic activity (the ECG may normalize after administering a beta-blocker), recent food ingestion, hyperventilation, ventricular hypertrophy, other cardiac anomalies (e.g. mitral valve prolapse).

Safety. The ECG must be continuously recorded and if the patient requests to stop the test should be terminated. If hypotension, arrhythmias or ST segment depression of greater than 2 mm develops, the test should be terminated. Providing care is taken to exclude patients with significant aortic stenosis, recent myocardial infarction or unstable angina and heart failure, then the risk of death or cardiac arrest is very low. Adequate resuscitation equipment and personnel skilled in resuscitation are mandatory.

Exercise testing in management of suspected angina

Use as a diagnostic test. The diagnosis of angina depends mainly on a careful history with emphasis on activities which precipitate or relieve symptoms. Whilst an abnormal ECG, e.g. inverted T waves, may support the diagnosis, severe ischaemia may be present in the context of a normal ECG at rest. There are serious limitations in the use of exercise testing in diagnosis, for instance development of ST depression during exercise may occur in some healthy subjects and especially in patients with mitral valve prolapse (false positive tests).

Conversely patients with significant coronary disease may not develop typical ST–T wave changes (false negative test), perhaps because the ischaemia is limited in extent or is remote from the chest wall (e.g. involving the posterior wall of the heart).

The value of any diagnostic test varies importantly according to the prevalence of the condition in the population under study. In the case of young women with atypical chest pain most of the patients showing exercise induced ST depression will not have cardiac ischaemia (poor specificity); conversely most 60 year old men with typical anginal symptoms will have coronary disease, although the exercise test will be positive in only a proportion (limited sensitivity). The value of the test depends on the pre-test probability of disease in the population being studied: if low, e.g. less than 10%, the test is of limited value and most of the abnormal tests will be due to a false positive.

Use as a prognostic test. All the variables measured during an exercise test may have value in predicting prognosis, for instance among middle aged men with angina those who complete Bruce stage III with a heart rate of greater than 140 beats per minute, a normal blood pressure response, without marked ST depression or arrhythmia, have an excellent outcome and a low prevalence of proximal multivessel coronary disease. In contrast patients with chest pain at stage I, with peak heart rate of less than 120 beats per minute or more than 1 mm ST depression, have a moderately high risk of clinical events (e.g. acute myocardial infarction or unstable angina may occur in 30% within 5 years); a high prevalence of these patients would have important coronary disease. Therefore, whilst exercise testing is limited as a diagnostic test it is highly useful as a prognostic test.

Exercise testing after acute myocardial infarction

Exercise testing is routine in many hospitals after recovery from an acute myocardial infarction (usually 1–4 weeks post infarct: a modified protocol to a lower peak heart rate is used). The test has some value in predicting patients who are likely to develop recurrent ischaemic events, e.g. unstable angina, post infarct angina, recurrent infarction, and is helpful in guiding rehabilitation. The prognosis after MI and especially the risk of sudden death relate more closely to the extent of myocardial damage and exercise testing is much less valuable in predicting early mortality (which is better predicted by measures of LV function, e.g. echocardiogram). However, patients who do develop clearcut ischaemia during the exercise test may need to be considered for early coronary angiography.

Exercise testing in other conditions

Heart failure. In patients with stable symptoms of heart failure, assessment of the workload and haemodynamic response (e.g blood pressure response) provide useful objective evidence of severity and may be valuable in measuring the response to treatment. Measurement of the oxygen uptake during exercise, which involves collection of expired gases, is very useful in predicting patients likely to deteriorate and is of value in selecting patients to be considered for cardiac transplant programmes.

Hypertrophic cardiomyopathy. Exercise testing is useful in determining the mechanism of syncope and in some patients may provoke arrhythmias, e.g. ventricular tachycardia, or demonstrate an abnormal haemodynamic response, e.g. hypotension due to left ventricular outflow tract obstruction, or abnormal vasoconstrictor response during exercise.

Suspected tachyarrhythmias. Both atrial (e.g. atrial fibrillation) and ventricular arrhythmias (e.g. ventricular tachycardia) may be provoked by exercise and this may help in the diagnosis and management by drug therapy.

Management of bradycardias. Children with congenital complete heart block may develop ventricular arrhythmias during exercise and this is a recognized indication for early pacemaker implantation. In patients with sick sinus syndrome and atrio-ventricular conduction disorders exercise testing may be useful to assess whether there is a normal increase in atrial rate during physical activity. This information may be used in deciding the choice of pacemaker prescription and in optimal adjustment of the pacemaker after implantation.

CARDIOVASCULAR MANIFESTATIONS OF SYSTEMIC DISEASE

The heart is affected in a variety of systemic disorders, including endocrine disorders, diabetes, connective tissue disease, infiltrations and neurological disease.

Endocrine disease

1. *Thyroid disease*
(a) *Hyperthyroidism.* The heart is very responsive to changes in thyroid hormone, and therefore cardiovascular symptoms and signs are important clinical features of hyperthyroidism. Palpitations, dyspnoea, systolic hypertension, tachycardia and a third heart sound are common. Sinus tachycardia occurs in 40% of patients with hyperthyroidism, and sustained atrial fibrillation in 20%. Atrial fibrillation in particular may be the only manifestation of hyperthyroidism. Other rhythm disturbances including atrioventricular (AV) block are seen less frequently. Both congestive cardiac failure and angina pectoris occur in hyperthyroid patients. The cardiac effects of hyperthyroidism respond well to beta-blockers (such as propranolol) but atrial fibrillation responds poorly to cardiac glycosides.
(b) *Hypothyroidism.* This can cause bradycardia, hypotension, congestive cardiac failure, hypercholesterolaemia, and pericardial effusion. Hypothyroidism can cause a cardiomyopathy, with dilated cardiac chambers and heart failure. Reversal of these abnormalities nearly always occurs with thyroid replacement therapy.

2. *Adrenal disease.* Cushing's syndrome (glucocorticoid excess) is associated with hypertension, hypercholesterolaemia and diabetes, and thus accelerated atherosclerosis. Addisons disease causes hypotension, often with marked postural accentuation. Sinus bradycardia is common. Although hyperkalaemia is frequently observed this rarely causes any cardiac toxicity. In primary hyperaldosteronism (Conn's syndrome)

hypertension, hypokalaemia and metabolic alkalosis are common.

Catecholamine-secreting tumours (phaeo-chromo-cytoma) often present with labile hypertension, but may also present with acute pulmonary oedema, paroxysmal arrhythmia or a myocarditic picture. The diagnosis is established by documenting increased plasma or urinary concentrations of catecholamines or their metabolites.

3. Acromegaly. Growth hormone excess is almost always characterized by cardiomegaly and left ventricular hypertrophy. Hypertension, premature ischaemic heart disease, cardiac failure, arrhythmias and insulin resistance are frequently found.

4. Carcinoid syndrome. Carcinoid tumours in the gut secrete serotonin, bradykinin and other humoral substances. The liver inactivates these substances, until liver metastases occur, when the systemic circulation is no longer protected from these substances. Cardiac manifestations include tricuspid and pulmonary stenosis or regurgitation. Mitral and aortic valve disease occurs rarely.

5. Diabetes. Cardiovascular disease is very common in diabetes, affecting both large and small vessels. This atherosclerosis tends to be more severe and more extensive than in non-diabetics. Lipid abnormalities, usually a mixed hyperlipidaemia, are common in diabetes. Insulin resistance contributes to the excess of coronary artery disease amongst Indo-Asians in Britain.

Not only is the severity of coronary artery disease and the frequency of coronary events increased in diabetics but the complication rate and mortality are also increased. Autonomic neuropathy is common, and thus pain perception in ischaemic heart disease is also affected. Diabetes increases the probability of developing cardiac failure, not only secondary to ischaemia but also due to a specific diabetic cardiomyopathy. Diabetes is also additive to atrial fibrillation for an increased risk of stroke and thromboembolism.

Connective tissue disease

1. Rheumatoid arthritis. Nodular granuloma can affect the myocardium and endocardium but rarely affects cardiac function. Pericarditis may be a presenting feature of rheumatoid arthritis, and is clinically diagnosed in 2% of patients with rheumatoid arthritis. Diffuse coronary arteritis also occurs but rarely results in myocardial ischaemia.

2. Systemic lupus erythematosus. Clinical evidence of pericarditis, myocarditis or endocarditis occurs in 50–60% of cases. Pericarditis is the most common manifestation and may cause effusion or constriction. Myocarditis often presents as left ventricular dysfunction, and severity is proportionate to that of the systemic disease. Libman–Sacks endocarditis can affect any part of the endocardium but rarely has functional consequences.

3. Ankylosing spondylitis. Aortic regurgitation, heart block and conduction disturbances relate to fibrous tissue deposition, which increases in frequency with disease duration. Cardiac dilatation and hypertrophy can also occur.

4. Marfan's syndrome. The most common cause of death is cardiovascular. Aortic wall degeneration leads to aortic root dilatation, dissecting aneurysms and aortic regurgitation. Mitral valve prolapse is also common.

Infiltrative disease

1. Haemochromatosis. This genetic disorder leads to deposition of iron in the heart, liver, pancreas and pituitary. Cardiac manifestations are cardiac failure and cardiac dilatation. Cardiac biopsy demonstrates the typical staining of excess iron deposition. Treatment is with phlebotomy or chelating agents.

2. Amyloidosis. Amyloidosis secondary to multiple myeloma frequently affects the heart, although secondary and familial forms may also do so, albeit less frequently. Restrictive cardiomyopathy is the most common manifestation, although systolic dysfunction, postural hypotension and conduction disturbances also occur. A speckled appearance of the left ventricular myocardium is the typical appearance on echocardiography. Diagnosis is by cardiac biopsy, although biopsy of non-cardiac sites (such as rectal mucosa, lymph nodes, etc.) often antedates the cardiac diagnosis.

3. Sarcoidosis. Cardiac sarcoid occurs in fewer than 5% of patients with sarcoidosis. This can present as cardiac failure (either congestive or restrictive in nature), conduction disturbances, ventricular arrhythmias, or sudden death. Cardiac biopsy may show the typical non-caseating granulomas. Management is difficult, although steroids may occasionally be of benefit.

Neurological disease

1. Muscular dystrophy. Duchennes muscular dystrophy frequently causes cardiac rhythm disturbances, and in the latter stages myocardial contractile dysfunction, although marked cardiac dilatation is unusual. Becker dystrophy affects all four cardiac chambers with ventricular dilatation and failure, in addition to frequent complete heart block. The rare Emery–Dreifuss dystrophy is associated with permanent atrial paralysis.

2. Freidreich's ataxia. Cardiac involvement although usually asymptomatic is very common, and frequently the cause of death in Freidreich's ataxia. A form of hypertrophic cardiomyopathy is most common, although a dilated cardiomyopathy with depressed systolic function is also seen.

3. Myotonic dystrophy. Cardiac involvement is concentrated predominantly on the His–Purkinje system, with a high frequency of AV and bundle branch block. Myocardial dystrophy is also seen, affecting all four cardiac chambers, although progression to overt heart failure is infrequent.

4. Guillain–Barre syndrome. Both brady- and tachy-arrhythmias are common, and if untreated can lead to sudden death. Autonomic instability can lead to profound changes in blood pressure and heart rate.

Further reading

Falk RH, Comenzo RL, Skinner M. The systemic amyloidoses. *New England Journal of Medicine.* 1997; **337:** 898–909.

CONGENITAL HEART DISEASE – AN INTRODUCTION

Congenital heart defects (CHD) occur in 0.6–0.8% of live births provided that there are no specific recognized risk factors, in which case this figure rises. The incidence increases to 2–3% if either parent or any siblings have CHD. First cousin marriages which are practised by some communities, carry a higher incidence than average of CHD especially those associated with heterotaxy (atrial isomerism) and complex heart defects. CHD are often diagnosed in early childhood although some remain unrecognized until adulthood. In the absence of symptoms, screening at birth and standard developmental check-ups at 6 weeks and 39 months often reveal the presence of CHD. Diagnosis is also possible antenatally for most defects, usually at around the 18th week of gestation, using ultrasound. Fetal echocardiography is indicated in high risk groups (e.g. positive family history, maternal diabetes, certain drugs, exposure to rubella, fetal arrhythmias and abnormal amniocentesis) or when a routine fetal scan fails to reveal normal cardiac anatomy. Some congenital defects which may avoid detection in childhood because of lack of symptoms or soft physical signs include atrial septal defect, coarctation, Ebstein's anomaly, divided left atrium (cor triatriatum) and congenitally corrected transposition.

Aetiology

Genetic

1. Chromosomal abnormality

- Extra chromosome e.g. Down's Syndrome.
- Deficient chromosome e.g. Turner's.
- Chromosome deletion e.g. Di George

2. Gene abnormality

- Syndrome
  i.   Dominant e.g. Marfan's.
  ii. Recessive e.g. Ellis van Creveld.
- Heart only
  i.   Dominant e.g. hypertrophic cardiomyopathy.
  ii. Recessive e.g. endocardial fibroelastosis.

Infections. Rubella (PDA, PA stenosis), cytomegalo virus.

Drugs. Phenytoin, lithium, alcohol.

Maternal problems. Diabetes mellitus, systemic lupus erythematosus.

Clinical presentation

Unless picked up antenatally, many patients with CHD present in early childhood either with heart failure, heart murmur, cyanosis or circulatory collapse.

Heart failure

- Large left to right shunts e.g. VSD, PDA, AVSD, large AV malformation
- Left sided stenotic lesions e.g. aortic stenosis, coarctation
- Valvar regurgitation e.g. aortic or mitral regurgitation
- Myocardial problems
  1. Metabolic: Pompe's Disease (hypertrophic cardiomyopathy), Acyl CoA dehydrogenase deficiency (dilated cardiomyopathy).
  2. Immunological: post viral, maternal SLE.
- Arrhythmias e.g. sustained paroxysmal supraventricular tachycardia, incessant tachycardia (permanent form of junctional reciprocating tachycardia), complete heart block.

Any of the above maybe present in combination.

Cyanosis

- Without heart failure
  1. Pulmonary atresia/ critical pulmonary stenosis.
  2. Severe Fallot.
  3. Severe tricuspid atresia with pulmonary stenosis/pulmonary atresia.
- With heart failure
  1. Transposition of great arteries.
  2. Hypoplastic left heart syndrome.
  3. Mixing of saturated with de-saturated blood.
     i.   At venous level e.g. total anomalous pulmonary venous drainage.
     ii. At atrial level e.g. common atrium.
     iii. At ventricular level e.g. single ventricle.

iv. At great artery level e.g. persistent arterial trunk

Although the presence of a heart murmur often directs attention to CHD, it is important to appreciate that some conditions may only have heart sounds. These include transposition, obstructed total anomalous pulmonary venous drainage, pulmonary atresia and coarctation.

Investigations

The electrocardiogram (ECG) provides helpful information regarding chamber hypertrophy and strain, axis and abnormalities of conduction. Lead V4R (mirror image of lead V4) provides useful information regarding right ventricular activity especially in infants.

The chest X-ray offers limited but useful information particularly with regards to heart size, heart shape and pulmonary vascularity.

The echocardiogram provides the most detailed information on cardiac morphology and function. When the trans-thoracic window is inadequate or gives incomplete information, trans-oesophageal echocardiography may prove very useful. The addition of colour and spectral Doppler offers qualitative and quantitative haemodynamic information.

Magnetic resonance imaging and spiral CT are also useful tools for non-invasive imaging although there are logistical limitations with these investigations.

Cardiac catheterization is performed less often nowadays for diagnostic purposes as ultrasound usually provides the information. It is, nevertheless, a useful adjunct to echocardiography for accurate assessment of haemodynamics, angiography as well as intervention.

Medical treatment for CHD

Overall care
- assessment
- fluid intake
- nutrition
- counselling

Drugs

- Heart failure: diuretics, ACE inhibitors, intravenous inotropes, Digoxin (for low output failure).
- PDA manipulation.
    1. Prostaglandin E1 or E2 (to maintain ductal patency).
    2. Indomethacin (for ductal closure).
- Myocardial contractility, beta blockers (Fallot/Marfan's Syndrome).

Rhythm therapy

- Anti-arrhythmic drugs.
- Pacing.
- Radiofrequency ablation for tachy-arrhythmias.

Intervention

- To replace surgery e.g. PDA\ASD closure.
- To complement surgery e.g. embolization of collaterals\atrial septostomy.

Surgery for CHD

- Palliative e.g. Blalock-Taussig shunt, cavo-pulmonary shunt, pulmonary artery band.
- Definitive palliative e.g.Fontan procedure.
- Reparative e.g. Fallot's repair, Rastelli procedure.
- Curative e.g. ASD closure.
- Transplantation e.g. heart or heart\lung or lung.
- Inoperable e.g. myocardial failure associated with generalized disorder.

Some conditions require a series of operations from any of the above categories.

Further reading

Neonatal Heart Disease. Eds. RM Freedom, LN Benson and JF Smallhorn. Springer-Verlag, Berlin, Heidelberg, New York, 1992.
Paediatric Cardiology. Eds. RH Anderson, FJ Macartney, EA Shinebourne and M Tynan. Churchill Livingston, Edindburgh, 1987.

CONGENITAL HEART DISEASE – ATRIAL SEPTAL DEFECT

This is a common defect forming around 10% of CHD. The commonest variety is the secundum ASD which is situated in the region of the oval fossa. On its own, it hardly ever gives rise to problems in infancy. Some 40% of secundum ASDs diagnosed in infancy are capable of spontaneous closure especially if they are less than 8 mm in diameter. In older patients, symptoms related to high output failure may become worse if atrial fibrillation sets in. Rarely, paradoxical embolization occurs in older patients.

Classical signs include right ventricular heave, ejection systolic murmur over the pulmonary area with some radiation to the back in the intra-scapular region as well as fixed splitting of the second heart sound. With large shunts, a low pitched diastolic murmur can be audible over the lower sternum arising from the tricuspid valve.

The ECG shows partial right bundle branch block with right axis deviation. The chest X-ray shows enlargement of the right atrium, right ventricle and pulmonary artery together with plethora but with a narrow pedicle. The echocardiogram shows right ventricular volume overload manifesting itself by a large right ventricle and paradoxical septal motion; it also demonstrates details of the defect and flow pattern on Doppler.

Traditionally, large atrial defects giving rise to a significant left to right shunt (often a 2:1 shunt is considered significant) have been surgically repaired with very good results and hardly any mortality or morbidity. Some 50% of these secundum defects can, nowadays, be closed with catheter techniques using double disc devices (e.g. ASDOS device) or self-centering joined discs (e.g. Amplatzer or Das Angel-Wing devices). Although most patients with significant ASDs are asymptomatic, improvement in exercise tolerance and well being as well as a reduction in chest infection rate occur following successful closure. In the long term, prevention of arrhythmias is an additional benefit.

There are two other types of ASDs which are numerically less common than the secundum type and for which surgery is required.

Partial atrio-ventricular septal defect

This was commonly referred to in the past as a primum ASD as it is associated with deficiency of the lower part of the inter-atrial septum close to the crux of the heart where the atrio-ventricular valves meet. There is absence of the atrio-ventricular septum and the two atrio-ventricular valves are, therefore, attached at the same level, unlike the normal situation where the tricuspid valve is attached closer to the apex of the heart. In this type of ASD, the ECG shows left axis deviation and is associated with a commissure in the septal leaflet of the mitral valve (sometimes referred to as 'cleft') and which can be responsible for mitral regurgitation resulting in left ventricular to right atrial shunting. The diagnosis is made by echocardiography and catheterization is not usually required. Surgical repair consists of patch closure of the defect and repair of the commissure in the mitral valve.

Sinus venosus defect

There are two types of this less common form of atrial septal defect depending on its position. More commonly, a venosus defect is situated in the upper part of the intra-atrial septum close to the entry of the superior vena cava to the right atrium. This type of venosus defect is often associated with anomalous drainage of the right pulmonary veins which either enter the right atrium or superior vena cava. The physical signs are similar to those found in a secundum ASD as are the ECG findings. The diagnosis is often made by precordial echocardiography although occasionally trans-oesophageal echocardiography may prove a superior tool particularly for identifying pulmonary venous drainage. Treatment is surgical with patch repair of the defect designed in a way to re-direct the pulmonary veins into the left atrium.

The second variety of venosus ASD is situated close to the inferior vena cava (IVC) as this vessel enters the right atrium. Occasionally, the IVC straddles the atrial septum and this may give rise to cyanosis. The physical signs, ECG and chest X-ray are similar as for a secundum ASD. Diagnosis is done on echocardiography with some advantage using trans-oesophageal echocardiogrpahy. Surgical repair involves insertion of a patch ensuring that the IVC drains into the right atrium.

A combination of the above types of atrial communications can co-exist and sometimes the atrial septum is fenestrated with several defects. The prognosis is excellent for all types of ASDs

although further mitral valve surgery maybe
required for the partial AVSD.

Further reading

Neonatal Heart Disease. Eds. RM Freedom, LN Benson and JF Smallhorn.
Springer-Verlag, Berlin, Heidelberg, New York, 1992.
Paediatric Cardiology. Eds. RH Anderson, FJ Macartney, EA Shinebourne and M
Tynan. Churchill Livingston, Edinburgh, 1987.

CONGENITAL HEART DISEASE – CYANOTIC CONDITIONS

Fallot's tetralogy

Fallot's Tetralogy consists of a combination of abnormalities, the four components in the original description being VSD, aortic override, right ventricular outflow obstruction and right ventricular hypertrophy. It is one of the commonest defects giving rise to cyanosis and forms around 10% of CHD. The main determinant of cyanosis is the degree of right ventricular outflow obstruction which often consists of subpulmonary or infundibular stenosis (caused by anterior and superior deviation of the outlet septum) as well as valvar stenosis; occasionally, there is also supra-valvar or pulmonary artery branch stenosis. If the degree of right ventricular outflow obstruction is mild, cyanosis may be minimal or absent and is referred to as 'acyanotic' Fallot. Variations or other associated abnormalities may be present in addition to the four basic abnormalities and these include ASD (known at Fallot's pentalogy), a right aortic arch (occurs in 25%), anomalous origin of coronary arteries, multiple ventricular septal defects, systemic collaterals from aorta to lungs or CAVSD (especially in Down's Syndrome).

When the right ventricular outflow tract obstruction is mild, the haemodynamics are consistent with a large left to right shunt and patients may present with symptoms of heart failure rather than cyanosis. The natural history is for the right ventricular obstruction to get progressively worse leading to worsening cyanosis. In toddlers, squatting is a classical manoeuvre to alleviate symptoms from cyanosis. Occasionally, cyanotic spells may lead to syncope and can be fatal. In addition to the cyanosis, there is usually a harsh ejection systolic murmur arising from the right ventricular outflow tract although this may become very quiet during a cyanotic spell.

The ECG shows right ventricular hypertrophy with right axis deviation although left axis may occur if there is an associated CAVSD. The chest X-ray shows typical uptilted apex with reduced vascularity and prominent pulmonary artery bay giving an appearance of a 'boot-shaped' heart. The echocardiogram is diagnostic but catheterization is often performed particularly to exclude multiple VSDs, to show coronary artery anatomy, to rule out collaterals arising from the aorta and to demonstrate the pulmonary artery anatomy within the lung parenchyma.

There is a role for medical treatment in cyanosed patients although ultimately surgery will be required. The use of beta blockers e.g. Propranolol improve cyanosis and reduce the incidence and severity of cyanotic spells. During a spell, treatment consists of placing the child over the shoulder in a knee-chest position, administration of oxygen, correction of metabolic acidosis, administration of morphine to reduce pain and tachypnoea, beta-blockers and, occasionally, Noradrenaline to increase the systemic vascular resistance.

Although balloon dilatation to the right ventricular outflow tract may improve cyanosis, this is only effective when the main component of the obstruction is at valvar or supra-valvar level but over 50% of the right ventricular obstruction is due to muscular obstruction in the subpulmonary region. Most patients are repairable with a one stage procedure but occasionally palliation may be required to improve cyanosis. There are two types of palliative procedures, 1. systemic to pulmonary artery shunt e.g. Blalock-Taussig shunt or 2. limited relief of right ventricular outflow tract obstruction by placement of patch and leaving the VSD intact. This is particularly used in small symptomatic infants with hypoplastic pulmonary arteries. Surgical repair is, however, preferable and possible in the majority and consists of patch repair of the ventricular septal defect and, nowadays, this is usually performed through a trans-atrial rather than a ventriculotomy approach where possible. In addition, the right ventricular outflow tract obstruction is relieved by resection of the muscular infundibular stenosis and enlargement of the pulmonary valve either by valvotomy or trans-annular patch if the pulmonary valve ring is small. Occasionally, it is necessary to use a conduit (prosthetic or homograft) between the right ventricle and pulmonary artery. Surgical mortality is between 3 and 5% and there is a 1–2% incidence of heart block requiring pacing.

Long-term prognosis is good although some will develop significant pulmonary regurgitation for which a valved conduit between the right ventricle and pulmonary artery will need to be inserted. Pulmonary regurgitation is generally very well tolerated and only a minority will require surgery and this is usually necessary several decades after the original repair. Late ventricular arrhythmias do occur partly related to surgery but also as part of the natural history of Fallot's Tetralogy. The trans-atrial approach not only carries haemodynamic benefits in the initial post-operative period but it is hoped that some late ventricular arrhythmias are also prevented.

Transposition of the great arteries

In the simple form, the aorta arises from the right ventricle and is anterior to the pulmonary artery which arises from the left ventricle. When associated with other abnormalities e.g. VSD, coarctation, pulmonary or subpulmonary stenosis, it is referred to as complex transposition. TGA forms around 5% of CHD and is three times more common in males.

Apart from cyanosis, these patients may have heart failure or present with circulatory collapse and metabolic acidosis. A loud second heart sound reflects the anteriorly placed aorta and murmurs may be present from VSD\PS when present.

The ECG shows right ventricular hypertrophy. The chest X-ray classically shows an 'egg-on-side' appearance with a narrow pedicle and sometimes pulmonary plethora or pulmonary venous congestion. The echocardiogram provides a definitive diagnosis including details of coronary artery anatomy which is useful for the current surgical method of treatment known as the arterial switch procedure.

In the absence of a good communication between the right and left side of the heart e.g. ASD\VSD\PDA, the degree of cyanosis can be severe. This can be alleviated by a simple procedure known as balloon atrial septostomy. This is performed under sedation by inserting a latex balloon catheter often through the umbilical vein, but occasionally through the femoral vein, into the left atrium and enlarging the foramen ovale by withdrawing the inflated balloon across the atrial septum into the right atrium. This can be performed under ultrasound control or alternatively by fluoroscopy. In addition, control of metabolic acidosis, diuretics and Prostaglandin may be required.

As the arterial switch operation initially carried a very high mortality, surgery consisted of atrial inflow operations designed to direct systemic and pulmonary venous blood to their physiologically appropriate great arteries. Two common types of such atrial inflow operations include the Mustard operation (where the atrium is divided using either prosthetic material or autologous pericardium) or the Senning operation in which the atria are re-arranged to achieve the same aim. These operations were often performed at between 6 and 12 months of age. The atrial switch operations have been replaced over the past decade by the arterial switch operation which is more physiological and which carries less than 5% mortality. In simple TGA, optimal timing is within the first 4 weeks of life, otherwise the left ventricle will not be able to sustained systemic workload. A recognized complication of the arterial switch is pulmonary branch stenosis which occurs in between 5 and 10% and which responds to balloon dilatation in round 60%.

In complex TGA, if there are other defects such as coarctation or ventricular septal defects, these are repaired at the same time as the arterial switch and the timing of surgery is similar to that for simple TGA although some do present later.

If complex TGA is associated with left ventricular outflow obstruction, usually in the form of pulmonary or subpulmonary stenosis, together with a ventricular septal defect, an initial palliative systemic to pulmonary artery shunt is performed to reduce the degree of cyanosis. An arterial switch is not usually possible and the operation of choice is an intra-ventricular repair consisting of patch closure of the VSD in such a way as to direct left ventricular flow to the aorta and using a conduit (prosthetic or homograft) between the right ventricle and pulmonary artery. This type of operation is referred to as the Rastelli procedure.

Some patients who have had the Mustard operation are now showing signs of severe right ventricular dysfunction usually with tricuspid regurgitation as, in this type of repair, the morphological right ventricle acts as a systemic ventricle. In some of these patients, a process to train the involuted left ventricle by applying a pulmonary artery band can be attempted. Those who respond appropriately to this mechanical afterload by hypertrophy and improved function can proceed to a late arterial switch and take-down of the inflow operation. Those who do not respond to the band or behave adversely can only benefit from transplantation.

Single ventricles

There are a number of conditions where there is only one functional ventricle, the other being either hypoplastic or replaced by a rudimentary chamber. Both mitral and tricuspid valves may enter the single ventricle (known as double inlet ventricle) or one of the AV valves may be atretic (tricuspid or mitral atresia).

Symptoms depend on the degree of pulmonary blood flow. If there is moderate reduction to pulmonary flow symptoms may be minimal. If there is severe reduction in pulmonary flow due to severe pulmonary stenosis or atresia of the pulmonary valve, cyanosis will be the predominant symptom. If, on the other hand, there is unrestrictive pulmonary flow, heart failure and/or pulmonary hypertension will be the presenting features.

The ECG is always abnormal depending on the underlying abnormality. The chest X-ray is also abnormal but features depend on the type of lesion, pulmonary flow and age at presentation. The echocardiogram is diagnostic although catheterization is usually necessary mainly to measure the pulmonary vascular resistance.

There is no cure for this group of conditions but palliative surgery helps. If there is reduced pulmonary blood flow a shunt will improve symptoms. If this is required in the first 3 months of life, a systemic to pulmonary artery shunt e.g. BT shunt, is usually performed by placing a Goretex tube of between 4 and 5 mm in diameter between the subclavian artery and the pulmonary artery. If the indication for surgery does not arise for a few months, a cavo-pulmonary shunt is preferable as this causes less volume loading on the single ventricle and lasts longer. If there is unrestricted flow to the pulmonary arteries, it is essential to protect the lungs from pulmonary vascular disease by placing a band across the main pulmonary artery. The ultimate procedure possible is a Fontan or total cavo-pulmonary connection (TCPC) which is a definitive palliative procedure designed to join the systemic veins directly into the pulmonary arteries bypassing the heart. The single ventricle acts as the systemic ventricle. This procedure can only be performed if certain criteria are met including a low pulmonary vascular resistance, good ventricular function and no significant valvar regurgitation. The Fontan operation is usually performed after the age of 3 years and sometimes in much older patients who have been previously palliated. Prognosis is good but guarded as some develop late failure due to reduced myocardial function and may require transplantation. Late arrhythmias are also common.

Congenital heart disease, even the very complex, is nowadays amenable to some form of intervention or surgery with most of the information obtainable by non-invasive methods.

Further reading

Neonatal Heart Disease. Eds. RM Freedom, LN Benson and JF Smallhorn. Springer-Verlag, Berlin, Heidelberg, New York, 1992.
Paediatric Cardiology. Eds. RH Anderson, FJ Macartney, EA Shinebourne and M Tynan. Churchill Livingston, Edinburgh, 1987.

CONGENITAL HEART DISEASE – MISCELLANEOUS ACYANOTIC CONDITIONS

Patent arterial duct (PDA)

Failure of the arterial duct to close spontaneously is a simple form of CHD. It results from a defect in the wall of the arterial duct and forms 10% of CHD, excluding PDA in premature infants. It is three times more common in females and may have a genetic aetiology in some cases.

A large PDA can give rise to heart failure, frequent chest infections and wheezing and can cause pulmonary hypertension. Apart from bounding pulses, there is a continuous murmur below the left clavicle and the left ventricualr apex maybe dynamic and displaced depending on the size of the shunt. When the duct is tiny or very large, only a systolic murmur maybe present.

The ECG maybe normal but may show left ventricular hypertrophy with large shunts. The chest X-ray shows cardiomegaly involving the left sided chambers together with plethora as well as broad pedicle. The echocardiogram demonstrates the duct as well as the degree of volume loading resulting from the shunt. Doppler shows continuous flow through the PDA and analysis of spectral Doppler can estimate pulmonary artery pressure.

A large PDA is common in very premature babies. In this group, administration of intravenous Indomethacin within the first 2 weeks of life may result in duct closure but this should only be given when clinically indicated e.g. uncontrollable heart failure or ventilator dependence due to large left to right shunt. If there is a contraindication to Indomethacin e.g. late symptoms, necrotizing enterocolitis, renal dysfunction or abnormal blood clotting, then surgical ligation is recommended and the earlier this is performed the quicker they can be weaned off the ventilator.

In babies born at term, a PDA does not usually give rise to uncontrollable heart failure and can be managed medically to give nature an opportunity to close it spontaneously or for the child to grow prior to closure. In most patients, nowadays, catheter closure is the preferred method even in older infants. Devices designed for this purpose include the Rashkind double umbrella or detachable coils (Duct Occlud or Cook PDA coils). The coils have the advantage of simplicity in deployment, smaller gauge tools, can be implanted through single vessel entry (femoral vein or artery) and are cheaper. If the duct is more than 9 mm in diameter, surgical ligation is often recommended although Nitinol-based devices currently being evaluated are likely to benefit larger ducts. There is a small incidence of residual shunt both following catheter closure and following surgical ligation and these are usually amenable to closure using coils. Long-term prognosis is excellent.

Atrio-ventricular septal defect (AVSD)

This condition is associated with absence of the atrio-ventricular septum which is situated at the crux of the heart between the insertion of the mitral and tricuspid valves. It forms 2–5% of CHD and is more common in Down's (contributing to 30% of CAVSD) compared to the normal population. When it involves the atrial septum only it is referred to as partial PAVSD and when the defect incorporates the lower part of the atrial septum and the inlet ventricular septum, it is referred to as complete AVSD (CVASD). There are intermediate types in between these two extremes. The AV valves are very abnormal often sharing a common orifice with bridging leaflets superiorly and inferiorly.

The symptoms are those of heart failure due to a large left to right shunt possibly with the addition of significant AV valve regurgitation. At birth, the heart may be silent but murmurs develop as pulmonary vascular resistance drops. The ECG shows right bundle branch block with a left or superior axis. There may be right or even left ventricular hypertrophy. There may also be a variable degree of AV block. The chest X-ray shows cardiomegaly with global cardiac enlargement and increased vascularity and a narrow pedicle. The echocardiogram is diagnostic and catheterization is often not required except when the pulmonary vascular resistance merits accurate measurement. In children with Down's Syndrome, many centres electively perform echocardiography on diagnosis of this syndrome, even in the absence of signs or symptoms, as the incidence of CHD is around 50%, with CAVSD being a common lesion.

Medical treatment for heart failure including diuretics and possibly ACE inhibitors. Surgery should be performed early, usually within the first 6 months of life, to prevent the onset of pulmonary hypertension especially in children with Down's Syndrome, who have additional reasons for developing pulmonary vascular disease, namely, upper airways obstruction due to small nostrils, large tonsils and adenoids and large tongue. There is very little scope for palliative surgery by banding the pulmonary artery and primary repair is preferred. Repair of CAVSD consists of repair of the defect using a two patch technique; a Dacron patch is used to close the ventricular component and a pericardial patch for the atrial component. The AV valves are also divided and repaired. In around 5%, the mitral valve needs to be replaced although this is not usually required at the time of the original operation. Surgical mortality is between 5 and 10% and this rises to between 15 and 20% when CAVSD is complicated by associated abnormalities such as double outlet right ventricle or Fallot's Tetralogy. There is a 5% risk of heart block needing pacing. The long-term outlook is good although some 10% will require further repair or replacement of the mitral valve usually many years following the original operation.

Pulmonary stenosis (PS)

Valvar PS as an isolated abnormality forms 5–8% of CHD.

Most are asymptomatic but have a prominent ejection systolic murmur over the pulmonary area with or without a click. When the degree of stenosis is critical, presentation may be in early infancy with cyanosis and may be duct dependent. Patients with Noonan's Syndrome commonly have pulmonary stenosis usually with a dysplastic pulmonary valve.

The ECG may show right axis deviation and right ventricular hypertrophy depending on the severity of the stenosis. When associated with Noonan's, the axis maybe leftward. The chest X-ray is usually normal but post stenotic dilatation may show a prominent pulmonary artery but with either normal or reduced vascularity. The echocardiogram confirms the diagnosis by showing thick pulmonary valve leaflets which do not open fully or may even show dysplastic leaflets. Doppler quantitates the gradient. Cardiac catheterization is only indicated if the gradient is considered significant (more than 50 mmHg) on Doppler and the procedure is performed largely to conduct balloon valvuloplasty which is successful in 95%. If the pulmonary valve is dysplastic, however, the results are less rewarding with some 40% requiring surgery for a valvotomy or excision of valve tissue possibly associated with a trans-annular patch.

Coarctation

Narrowing of the upper thoracic aorta beyond the left subclavian artery is twice as common in males and forms between 5 and 8% of CHD. Although often it is an isolated problem it can be associated with other defects including shunts e.g. VSD\AVSD or left ventricular outflow obstruction e.g. aortic stenosis\discrete subaortic stenosis\aortic arch hypoplastia.

Clinically, presentation can occur in early infancy with heart failure, circulatory collapse or metabolic acidosis and, in this group, the coarctation is usually situated proximal to the PDA i.e. pre-ductal or across the PDA i.e. juxta-ductal. The mechanism is a sling of ductal tissue surrounding the descending aorta and causing stenosis as the duct closes. Alternatively, presentation can occur later on in life, sometimes even in adulthood, with hypertension, reduced femoral pulses, aortic regurgitation or heart failure. In this group the narrowing is usually post-ductal.

Examination reveals absent or weak femoral pulses with radio-femoral delay and possibly hypertension. There may not be any murmurs but bruits can be heard over the left scapula in older patients once significant collaterals have developed.

The ECG shows right ventricular hypertrophy in the infant presentation but may be normal or show left ventricular hypertrophy in the post-ductal variety. The chest X-ray shows cardiomegaly and pulmonary oedema for the pre-ductal coarctation but may be normal or show a left ventricular contour in the post-ductal type. In addition, the ascending aorta is prominent and there may be an indentation in the upper thoracic aorta giving rise to a 'figure of three' appearance. Rib notching may occur but not usually before the age of 6 years. The echocardiogram is diagnostic in infants but maybe less informative in older patients due to a poor supra-sternal window. The Doppler pattern is diagnostic showing a high V_{max} in the descending aorta accompanied by a diastolic slope caused by failure of pressure to equalize across the stenosis. If a coarctation cannot be seen at the usual site, it is worth bearing in mind the possibility of coarctation in the lower thoracic aorta (sometimes associated with neurofibromatosis) or involving the abdominal aorta. An MRI scan helps identify the lesion when an echocardiogram is inconclusive.

Coarctation presenting in early infancy is usually an emergency. Initial medical treatment consists of correcting metabolic acidosis, diuretics, fluid restriction, inotropes and Prostaglandin to encourage ductal patency. Although balloon dilatation is sometimes effective in this group, there is a high recurrence rate of around 30% together with damage to the femoral artery from the balloon. Surgery, therefore, is preferred for pre-ductal coarctation and it consists of resection of the coarctation with end to end anastomosis; alternatively a left subclavian flap aortoplasty or patch aortoplasty can be performed also through a left thoracotomy. When there is an associated large ventricular septal defect one option is to repair the coarctation and place a pulmonary artery band to protect the pulmonary arteries and control heart failure, followed by de-band and repair of VSD at a later date. Alternatively, and this is our preferred approach, the coarctation and ventricular septal defect are repaired at the same session through a median sternotomy using circulatory arrest and deep hypothermia.

In older patients presenting with coarctation or in the event of post-surgical re-coarctation, balloon dilatation is the treatment of choice. There is around 10% recurrence both following surgery and balloon dilatation. So long as the balloon size does not exceed the diameter of the narrowest native aorta, the risk of aneurysm formation or rupture is very low indeed. The prognosis is good but these patients require long-term follow-up.

Further reading

Neonatal Heart Disease. Eds. RM Freedom, LN Benson and JF Smallhorn. Springer-Verlag, Berlin, Heidelberg, New York, 1992.
Paediatric Cardiology. Eds. RH Anderson, FJ Macartney, EA Shinebourne and M Tynan. Churchill Livingston, Edinburgh, 1987.

CONGENITAL HEART DISEASE – VENTRICULAR SEPTAL DEFECT

This is the commonest form of CHD and forms around 25% of all defects.

VSDs come in different sizes, small ones often close spontaneously within the first 5 years of life. Larger ones may become smaller and even close spontaneously but generally require surgery either because of heart failure, elevation of pulmonary artery pressure or haemodynamically significant shunt. If surgery is not required for these reasons within the first 2 years of life, it may still be indicated because of increase in left ventricular volume overload, onset of aortic regurgitation or bacterial endocarditis. Spontaneous closure of VSD is sometimes associated with the development of a discrete fibrous membrane below the aortic valve involving the ventricular septum and septal leaflet of the mitral valve and which can lead to progressive left ventricular outflow obstruction as well as aortic regurgitation.

VSDs can occur anywhere on the ventricular septum but the majority are situated in the region of the membranous septum. Other sites include the inlet, the outlet or the muscular portions of the septum and when these types of defects are adjacent to the membranous septum they are referred to as peri-membranous; hence, peri-outlet VSD if extending to the outlet septum. An unusual type of outlet VSD is associated with absence of the outlet septum resulting in continuity between the aortic and pulmonary valves and the defect is, therefore, situated directly underneath both great arteries; this is referred to as doubly committed or supracristal VSD. These defects can be associated with a high pulmonary artery flow and may look deceptively small. As the aortic valve is unsupported it may prolapse and lead to regurgitation. There may be malalignment of the aorta with the ventricular septum in some patients with outlet VSDs; this appearance is known as aortic override, the degree of which can be variable. Although aortic override may be present in isolated defect, it is more common in complex anomalies such as Fallot's Tetralogy or persistent arterial trunk.

Clinical signs include a harsh, uniformly pan-systolic murmur heard all over the precordium and which may be accompanied by a thrill. The presence of a dynamic displaced apex and a mitral diastolic flow murmur indicate the presence of a large shunt. A loud pulmonary second heart sound is ominous especially if accompanied by a reduction in the murmur as this reflects the onset of pulmonary vascular disease.

The ECG shows left ventricular hypertrophy initially with voltage changes in the central chest leads but later also involving the lateral leads. The chest X-ray shows cardiac enlargement involving the left atrium and left ventricle together with plethora but with a narrow pedicle. The definitive diagnosis is made on echocardiography where the site, size and number of defects can be made as well as an assessment of left ventricular volume overload as judged by the ratio of the aorta to left atrium as well as left ventricular dimension in diastole. A VSD which is more than two thirds the size of the aortic root is usually haemodynamically significant. Spectral Doppler helps in the assessment of right ventricular pressure, so long as there is no right or left ventricular outflow obstruction, by measuring the maximal velocity across the VSD. In addition, the right ventricular pressure can be estimated from the tricuspid regurgitant jet; if this is elevated it is essential to distinguish between associated right ventricular outflow tract obstruction or pulmonary hypertension by measuring the velocity across the pulmonary valve. Colour Doppler is very useful to pick up muscular defects which may not be easily apparent on cross-sectional echocardiography because of the septal trabeculations. Cardiac catheterization maybe required if the pulmonary vascular resistance is elevated, if other abnormalities are suspected or if multiple defects need clarification.

Medical treatment is of limited value and consists of treatment of heart failure and optimizing nutrition. Although some VSDs have been closed through catheter techniques, the treatment is largely surgical. Repair should be performed using a patch rather than direct suture as the latter is very often associated with residual shunts. The preferred current surgical method is through a trans-atrial approach thus avoiding a ventriculotomy with its potential problems of right ventricular dysfunction and ventricular tachy-arrhythmias. Repair, even in infancy, carries less than 3% risk with a rare but recognized incidence of heart block of round 1% for which pacing is required. Long-term prognosis is excellent.

Further reading

Neonatal Heart Disease. Eds. RM Freedom, LN Benson and JF Smallhorn. Springer-Verlag, Berlin, Heidelberg, New York, 1992.
Paediatric Cardiology. Eds. RH Anderson, FJ Macartney, EA Shinebourne and M Tynan. Churchill Livingston, Edinburgh, 1987.

DISEASES OF THE PERICARDIUM

Acute /inflammatory pericarditis

This usually presents with a sharp, constant sternal pain radiating to the left shoulder, sometimes down the arm. The pain is classically made worse by breathing, coughing and lying to the left and the back, and is usually relieved by sitting up. A pericardial friction rub, which is usually best heard at the left sternal edge, is the diagnostic sign. The ECG shows diffuse convex ST segment elevation except in lead aVR, with upright T-waves and without reciprocal changes. The CXR is usually normal unless there is a significant pericardial effusion.

Acute pericarditis is mostly viral in nature (Coxsackie), but it may be caused by other infections such as tuberculosis or other bacterial infections. Connective tissue disease, acute myocardial infarction, malignancy, trauma, Dressler's syndrome, uraemia and radiotherapy are other causes. Pericarditis may be also caused by drugs such as hydralazine, procainamide or practolol. Hypothyroidism is an unusual cause of pericardial effusion.

Non-steroidal anti-inflammatory agents are useful to control pain. In some patients, the condition may be recurrent, possibly due to an immunological abnormality, that causes recurrent attacks of pericarditis. Such cases can be treated by anti-inflammatory agents, including aspirin, colchicine, prednisolone or azathioprine. Pericardiotomy may rarely be required.

Pericardial effusion

The commonest causes are infection (e.g. viral, TB), and neoplasm. The most common cancers are breast, lymphoma or bronchogenic. AIDS may dispose to opportunistic infection.

There are no specific signs unless there is pericardial tamponade. Venous pressure is usually elevated and the CXR shows cardiomegaly. Diagnosis is confirmed by the presence of an echo-free area in front of the right ventricle and behind the left ventricle. Unless the fluid accumulates very quickly, small effusions (<1cm) do not need intervention.

The patient is observed for the development of any symptoms, increasing dyspnoea, cough and malaise, and signs of haemodynamic compromise such as tachycardia, pulsus paradoxus (a fall in systolic pressure >10mmHg on spontaneous inspiration), hypotension, elevated venous pressure and declining urine output.

Diuretics should be avoided and fluids may be needed to increase cardiac filling pressures. If the condition worsens, pericardiocentesis is required which will be both therapeutic and diagnostic (fluid is sent for bacteriology, biochemisty, histology and haematocrit). Regardless of the cause, pericardial fluid is mostly haemorrhagic. Draining a small amount might be enough to relieve the patient's distress and the drain might be left *in situ* for 24 hours or longer until echocardiography confirms the near-complete clearance of fluid. Balloon pericardiotomy may be indicated for recurrent malignant effusion.

Cardiac tamponade

The diagnosis of tamponade should be considered in any patient with a low output state, high venous pressure (characterized by a dominant x descent coincident with the carotid pulse) and oliguria. The rapid accumulation of pericardial fluid interferes with the diastolic filling of both left and right ventricles resulting in elevation of their diastolic pressures. Pulsus paradoxus is present in most cases, except in aortic regurgitation, atrial septal defect and uraemic patients undergoing haemodialysis due to elevated left ventricular diastolic pressure.

Echocardiographic examination must be performed even if the heart is small in size, as it might be in acute traumatic cases with previously normal hearts. Right atrial compression and collapse of the right ventricle in diastole are diagnostic of tamponade on echocardiography.

All significantly compromised patients must undergo pericardiocentesis or open drainage.

Constrictive pericarditis

Volume infusions might provide temporary supportive treatment. Patients with small effusions (<1cm) should be observed and closely monitored (including serial echocardiograms) while receiving anti-inflammatory treatment.

Constrictive pericarditis has the same pathophysiological features as pericardial tamponade in terms of impaired diastolic filling. However, there is no pulsus paradoxus and the venous pressure shows rapid y descent, which is out of phase with the carotid pulse. The symptoms and signs are generally similar to severe right ventricular failure (with severe oedema, ascites and hepatomegaly) with an impalpable apex and a third heart sound ('pericardial knock'). The ECG shows non-specific ST/T wave changes. Chest X-ray or CT scan may show pericardial calcification. The right and left ventricular pressures show equalization (± 5 mmHg), and a 'dip and plateau' (square root) configuration.

The common causes are previous TB, radiation, previous cardiac surgery and SLE. The differential diagnosis includes liver cirrhosis (normal venous pressure), tricuspid valve disease, right ventricular infarct (features of ischaemic heart disease present) and restrictive cardiomyopathy (no calcification, square root diastolic pressure sign that is significantly higher in the left ventricle, but biopsy is sometimes needed to differentiate). Pericardiectomy is performed when the diagnosis is confirmed.

Effusive constrictive pericarditis occurs when there is pericardial effusion, often with tamponade, and pericardial pathology. Drainage of pericardial fluid reveals the clinical and haemodynamic features of constrictive pericarditis.

Dressler's (post-pericardiotomy syndrome)

This syndrome is probably autoimmune in nature. It may appear a week or two post-myocardial infarction or cardiac surgery and is sometimes delayed and recurrent. In rare occasions, it may be the first presentation of a previously silent MI. There is fever and leucocytosis. Anti-inflammatory drugs ±

prednisolone should be used; drainage is seldom necessary.

Tuberculosis pericarditis

It should be suspected in immunosuppressed patients, such as in AIDS and haemodialysis subjects, as well as if no obvious aetiology was found or if there was no response to standard anti-inflammatory agents. It is usually treated by triple therapy ± prednisolone.

Collagen disease induced pericarditis

Fibrinous pericarditis develops in many patients with lupus erythematosus. Secondary bacterial infection might appear due to immunosuppression. Tamponade and constrictive pericarditis may develop.

Rheumatoid arthritis can cause subacute constrictive pericarditis with other features such as heart block and valve disease. Pericardiectomy is often needed.

Neoplastic involvement of the pericardium

Commonly, this is due to secondary deposits, as mentioned above. Mesothelioma is a very rare primary tumour. Cardiac tamponade is the commonest complication.

Radiation induced pericardial disease

Mediastinal radiation can result in early or late constrictive pericarditis or restrictive cardiomyopathy. Pericardiectomy might be useful if the latter is excluded by endomyocardial biopsy.

HYPERTENSION

High blood pressure affects around 7.5 million people in England and Wales and is, therefore, the most common chronic medical condition. There is, however, good evidence that the management of hypertension is of a very low standard with high levels of under-diagnosis and under-treatment as well as some over-treatment.

Definition

High blood pressure is difficult to define because there is a close linear relationship between the height of the systolic and diastolic blood pressure and the subsequent development of both heart attacks and stroke. This relationship continues within the so-called normal range so that an individual with a diastolic blood pressure of 85 mmHg is at greater risk than a similar individual with a pressure of 75 mmHg. For this reason, a good criterion for diagnosing hypertension is to take that level of blood pressure where investigation and treatment have been shown to do more good than harm. This therapeutic definition of hypertension is dependent on the results of randomized controlled trials many of which were published since 1990. Current evidence suggests that hypertension should be defined as a systolic blood pressure of greater than 140–160 mmHg and a diastolic pressure of greater than 90–95 mmHg.

Prevalence of hypertension The prevalence of hypertension in a population depends on the age distribution and the number of blood pressure readings taken. Over the age of 80, blood pressures of 160/95 or more are seen in approximately 50% of the population. Among 45–64-year-old men and women in Renfrew, Scotland, diastolic blood pressures of greater than 90 mmHg were found in 25% of the population. Thus hypertension becomes more common with advancing age and this was once considered to be a 'normal' phenomenon. More recently it has been shown that the rise in blood pressure with age, associated with a rise in the prevalence of hypertension, is only seen in societies which have a high dietary salt intake.

There is evidence from the USA that hypertension is roughly twice as common in blacks compared to white people. Figures in Britain are similar although perhaps not so extreme. There is no convincing evidence that black people consume more salt than white people although they may be more sensitive to a given salt load.

Complications of hypertension

Hypertension is one of three risk factors for premature heart attack and stroke. For coronary heart disease, high blood cholesterol and cigarette smoking are synergistic risk factors which when present have a multiplicative effect on the risk of death. With stroke disease, high blood pressure is the primary risk factor with cigarette smoking being important particularly for cerebral and sub-arachnoid haemorrhage. The relationship between serum cholesterol and stroke is weak and may be only effective over a long period.

When assessing hypertensive patients, it is important to assess their total cardiovascular risk taking into account all three risk factors. If for a given level of blood pressure there is also left ventricular hypertrophy, then the risk can be multiplied by three-fold and similarly diabetes exerts a very powerful effect.

At a clinical level, malignant phase hypertension if left untreated is associated with an 88% 2-year mortality rate. A diastolic blood pressure of 120 mmHg on its own is associated with a 16% 2-year mortality if left untreated. Among milder degrees of hypertension, epidemiological evidence shows that blood pressure of 150/100 mmHg at the age of 35 is associated with a $16^1/_2$ year reduction in life expectancy with death due to heart attack and stroke.

High blood pressure is an underlying cause of heart failure being responsible for 70% of cases. It is also seen in about 30% of patients with peripheral vascular disease. High blood pressure is also a cause of chronic renal failure; most patients with intrinsic renal disease have high blood pressure which in turn causes further renal damage. There remains, however, some doubt as to whether high blood pressure can affect the undamaged kidney in the same way as it can affect the undamaged heart or brain.

Recent evidence suggests that high blood pressure is associated with both multi-infarct dementia and Alzheimer's disease and these findings are backed up by the observation that antihypertensive therapy appears to be associated with some improvement in cerebral function.

The aetiology of hypertension

The number of people with abnormal blood pressure is directly proportional to the average blood pressure of the population. Thus, when investigating the aetiology of hypertension, one has to look at factors affecting the blood pressure of the population as a whole. The multinational INTERSALT project clearly demonstrated that obesity, a high salt intake and a high alcohol intake were all associated with raised blood pressure and the rise in blood pressure with age. These factors may act in association with hereditary factors. Studies of mono- and dizygotic twins as well as adopted and non-adopted children strongly suggest a powerful genetic inheritance.

Underlying diseases which cause high blood pressure ('secondary hypertension') are seen in between 2 and 5% of hypertensives, depending on the criteria for diagnosis. These include phaeochromocytoma, tumorous hyperaldosteronism (Conn's syndrome) and non-tumorous hyperaldosteronism, coarctation of the aorta, renal artery stenosis (fibro-muscular hyperplasia or atheroma), Cushing's syndrome and intrinsic renal diseases. All renal diseases are associated with hypertension but IgA nephropathy and polycystic disease are particularly closely associated. Almost all patients with chronic renal failure have hypertension. Hypertension is strongly associated with both non-insulin-dependent and insulin-dependent diabetes mellitus and is intimately linked with hyperlipidaemia. These associations may be related to common aetiology related to insulin resistance.

Mechanisms of hypertension

High blood pressure is related to the interplay between the activity of the renin angiotensin system and body fluid volume. These factors both operate even when absolute levels of renin and total body sodium are within the normal range. There is now evidence that non-circulating renin angiotensin systems play an important role in the pathogenesis of high blood pressure as well as the development of left ventricular hypertrophy and hypertension-associated renal damage.

The sympathetic nervous system is also implicated in the pathogenesis of hypertension particularly in relation to day-to-day variability in blood pressure. There is, however, little convincing evidence that stress itself plays any role in the pathogenesis of hypertension although it may be associated with falsely elevated blood pressures in anxious individuals.

Many other neurohumoral mechanisms have been implicated in the pathogenesis of hypertension but their roles are uncertain. These include the kalikrein kinin system, the endothelins, medullophilins, ouabain and intracellular calcium levels.

Blood pressure measurement

The optimal method of measuring blood pressure is as employed in the randomized controlled trials. Blood pressures should normally be measured seated with the arm cuff at the same level as the heart. The column of mercury should be deflated at 2–3 mm/s and blood pressures recorded to the nearest 2 mmHg. Blood pressures should be measured twice at each consultation. Standing blood pressures need only be measured for people with postural symptoms. Diastolic blood pressures should be measured in both pregnant and non-pregnant women at phase 5 (disappearance of sounds). There is reliable evidence that the quality of blood pressure measurement by doctors and the quality of assessment of hypertensive patients is very bad. The value of 24-hour ambulatory blood pressure monitoring is controversial and may not be more predictive than reliable assessment by well trained doctors and nurses in the clinical environment. Nevertheless some patients do exhibit a marked white coat effect. This state should be suspected in people with high blood pressure who have no evidence of end organ damage and no left ventricular hypertrophy (LVH) on their ECG. There is now evidence that patients whose blood pressures are raised in the clinical environment but normal under home conditions are at intermediate risk between those with persistently normal pressures and those with sustained hypertension although their clinical management remains uncertain.

The investigation of hypertension

In most hypertensive patients, the only investigations that are necessary are routine dipstix testing of the urine, estimation of serum creatinine and electrolytes, plasma cholesterol and an ECG. More detailed investigation is only necessary in very young patients or in those where the preliminary investigations or the clinical history suggest an underlying cause for high blood pressure. Patients with paroxysmal hypertension associated with tachycardia, blanching and weight loss should undergo a 24-hour urine collection for catecholamines to exclude phaeochromocytoma. Patients with an unprovoked serum potassium of below 3.6, particularly if the serum sodium is greater than 140, should undergo estimation of renin and aldosterone levels. If the femoral, dorsalis pedis or posterior tibial pulses are weak or delayed, patients should have their blood pressure measured, using a large cuff, in their legs and where necessary referred for cardiological investigation to exclude coarctation of the aorta. Patients with renal impairment or proteinuria should undergo ultrasonography of the kidneys. Renal arteriography should be conducted in patients with evidence of peripheral vascular disease, abdominal bruits and an over-rapid response to ACE inhibitors or asymmetrical kidney size on ultrasonography.

The value of antihypertensive treatment

Antihypertensive treatment is effective in preventing both heart attacks and strokes. A recent meta-analysis of all clinical trials shows that the control of blood pressure is associated with a 38% reduction of stroke and a 16% reduction of coronary heart disease. There is also evidence that the control of blood pressure can delay renal failure in patients with renal impairment.

The treatment of hypertension in the elderly is particularly worthwhile and therapy has been validated up to the age of 80 years. In older people, it has been shown that the treatment of isolated systolic hypertension (systolic blood pressure greater than 160 mmHg and diastolic blood pressure below 90 mmHg) is effective in preventing both heart attacks and strokes. Isolated systolic hypertension in the elderly, once thought to be a benign condition, is now known to be well worth treating.

Choice of antihypertensive drug

Only the beta blockers and the thiazides have been shown, in randomized controlled trials, to prevent heart attacks and strokes, and are therefore classed as first line agents. The newer agents such as calcium antagonists, ACE inhibitors and alpha blockers have been classed by the British Hypertension Society guidelines (1992) as 'alternative' first line agents.

The newer classes of drug have not been subjected to such trials and more information should become available by the year 2000. The ACE inhibitors have, however, been shown to be superior to other classes of drugs in reducing left ventricular hypertrophy and proteinuria and to delay renal deterioration in diabetics and non-diabetics with renal damage. There remains a question over the safety of the dihydropyridine calcium channel blockers in patients with existing coronary heart disease, with some evidence for an adverse effect from using the short-acting dihydropyridines, such as nifedipine capsules. Nevertheless, data from the recent SYST-EUR study, with the dihydropyridine calcium antagonist, nitrendipine, have been very reassuring, with a reduction in mortality, strokes and cardiac events, and no significant excess of malignancy or bleeding. The relative benefits of the alpha receptor blockers (prazosin, doxazosin) and of the angiotensin II receptor blockers (losartan, valsartan, irbesartan) remain uncertain.

Drugs which work wholly or in part by blocking the renin angiotensin system tend to be less effective in patients where plasma renin levels are low. Low plasma renin levels are seen in older patients and in Afro-Caribbeans. This explains why the beta blockers and the ACE inhibitors are less effective in these groups of patients. The thiazide diuretics or long-acting calcium channel blockers are the preferred option.

When a second antihypertensive agent is introduced, the choice should be of one where synergism in action has been demonstrated, for example, ACE inhibitors and diuretics, beta blockers and calcium antagonists, etc. Co-morbidity also has to be considered, for example, a hypertensive patient with angina may benefit from beta blockers or calcium antagonists, while if concurrent heart failure is present, ACE inhibitors and diuretics are the sensible choice. However, in diabetic patients, the use of thiazides may worsen diabetic control and excerbate hyperlipidaemia. Individual drug side-effects have to be considered for the individual patients. For example, use of thiazides and beta blockers in the young may result in impotence, while ACE inhibitors have cough as a significant side-effect.

When effectively applied, non-pharmacological methods of reducing blood pressure are useful at controlling blood pressure and are about as effective as any single drug therapy. All hypertensive patients should be instructed to reduce their salt intake to below 100 mmol per day and where relevant, to reduce their alcohol intake and lose weight. Weight loss is associated with an approximate 1 mmHg per kg reduction in blood pressure. All patients with hypertension should be counselled intensively on non-drug therapies.

In patients recovering from a stroke, antihypertensive treatment is best withheld in the acute stages. On a long-term basis, the control of severe hypertension is associated with reduction of stroke recurrence but its value in the treatment of mild post stroke hypertension remains uncertain. Following a MI, there is evidence that in hypertensives and normotensives, the beta blockers, the ACE inhibitors and verapamil are associated with a reduction of reinfarction rates. The control of blood pressure has been shown to ameliorate heart failure and reduce angina. At the present state of knowledge, the clinician should aim to reduce the blood pressure to below 160/90 mmHg, possibly with more aggressive management in patients who also have diabetes or renal impairment.

Further reading

Collins R, MacMahon S. Blood pressure, antihypertensive drug treatment and the risks of stroke and coronary heart disease. *British Medical Bulletin,* 1994; **50:** 272–98.

Dodson PM, Lip GYH, Eames SM, Gibson JM, Beevers DG. Hypertensive retinopathy: a review of existing classification systems and a suggestion for a simplified grading system. *Journal of Human Hypertension,* 1996; **10:** 93–8.

O'Brien, Beevers DG, Marshall H. *ABC of Hypertension.* London: BMJ Publications, 1996.

Joint National Committee on Detection, Evaluation and Treatment of High Blood Pressure. The Fifth Report of the Joint National Committee on Detection, Evaluation and Treatment of High Blood Pressure (JNC V). *Archives of Internal Medicine,* 1993; **153:** 154–83.

Sever P, Beevers G, Bulpitt C, Lever A, Ramsay L, Reid J, Swales J. Management guidelines in essential hypertension: report of the second working party of the British Hypertension Society. *British Medical Journal,* 1993; **306:** 983–7.

INFECTIVE ENDOCARDITIS

Definition

Infective endocarditis (IE) implies bacterial or fungal infection of intracardiac tissue. Acute and subacute presentations are recognized depending on the clinical profile and expected progression in the absence of medical therapy. Acute IE is typically associated with rapid valve destruction, widespread metastatic abscesses and rapidly fatal outcome (usually within 6 weeks). Subacute infection usually affects anatomically abnormal valves and may have an indolent downhill course of several months. Metastatic abscesses are uncommon presentations. In the era of antibiotics and surgery, classical presentations are rare. For example, infection of native 'normal' valves is unusual, unless patients are intravenous drug abusers or have mitral valve prolapse; by contrast, prosthetic valve infection may occasionally occur.

Native valve endocarditis Pre-existent cardiac lesions are present in 60–80% of patients.

1. Congenital heart disease. Ventricular septal defect (VSD), patent ductus arteriosus, aortic and pulmonary stenosis are the most common predisposing congenital diseases but early corrective surgery reduces risk. Many small VSDs are managed conservatively and are susceptible to IE both at the site of defect and at the site of impingement of the trans-VSD jet in the right ventricle. Residual VSDs and valve inadequacies after corrective surgery are also susceptible. Isolated ostium secundum atrial septal defects (ASD) are however seldom affected because of low turbulence and pressures. Primum ASDs are associated with mitral leaflet clefts which are susceptible to IE affecting this valve.

The most common organisms in children are *Streptococcus viridans* and Group D streptococci but the incidence of *Staphylococcus aureus* is increasing.

A bicuspid aortic valve is an important predisposing cause in older men where these valves have calcified and stenosed or become incompetent. Aortic coarctation is associated with a risk of endarteritis at the coarct site and at the commonly associated bicuspid aortic valve.

2. Rheumatic valve disease. Rheumatic valve involvement has declined in the developed countries in the last 40 years and is usually seen in the elderly and immigrants. In general the mitral valve tends to be the most common site for IE, followed by the aortic. Tricuspid and pulmonary valve involvement is rare.

3. Mitral valve prolapse. Mitral valve prolapse is common in young adults (prevalence 2–5% in young populations; up to 20% in young women in some series). The likelihood of IE is greatest if the prolapsing valve is also regurgitant (0.52 per 1000 patient years) and tends to be highest in older patients and males. The risk in uncomplicated prolapse (0.046 per 1000 patient years) is not significantly different from the population in general.

4. Hypertrophic obstructive cardiomyopathy. Predisposes to IE especially where the systolic gradient is high. Vegetations can form at the aortic valve, mitral leaflets or subaortic endothelium, all of which are subject to kinetic stress in this condition.

5. Marfan's syndrome. If associated with aortic incompetence Marfan's syndrome predisposes to IE of the anterior mitral leaflet where the jet impinges rather than the aortic valve itself.

6. Degenerative valve disease. An increasing incidence of IE is being seen in the elderly with degenerative valve disease, for example, aortic sclerosis, where the aortic valve is thickened and irregular.

7. Endocarditis in intravenous drug abusers. Incidence varies with injection habit (e.g. syringe cleanliness) and drug being injected: for example, cocaine use is less often associated with IE than the use of heroin and amphetamines. Even successfully treated individuals are more prone to re-infection. The tricuspid valve is involved in about half. Half have aortic or mitral involvement, and multiple valve infections are not uncommon. Pulmonary involvement is being increasingly recognized with development of transoesophageal echocardiography.

Right-sided endocarditis may present as pneumonia or septic pulmonary emboli and parasternal murmurs in these individuals should not be automatically labelled as 'functional'. Involvement of the tricuspid valve can present as torrential tricuspid regurgitation, especially if there is a flail valve leaflet.

Most bacterial isolates are skin commensals, but some are contaminants of drugs and injection devices. *S. aureus* is isolated in 60%, various streptococci and enterococci in 20%, Gram-negative bacilli in 10%, and fungi and *Candida* in 5%. Anaerobes are uncommon but should be suspected in persistently culture negative situations. Mixed isolates occur in 95% of cases.

8. Prosthetic valve endocarditis. Approximately 5% of prosthetic valve recipients develop IE within 10 years of implant, the risk being highest in the early period after surgery. Infection developing in the first 2 months after surgery differs from that occurring afterwards and usually reflects perioperative contamination. *S. aureus* and *S. epidermidis,* often methicillin-resistant, are the most common (25–30% of each) isolates but fungi and anaerobes are sometimes seen.

Currently there seems to be no difference in predisposition to infection between metal and tissue valves.

Pathogenesis

Flow impact, bacterial adhesivness, endothelial denudation and clot-cascade activation are of importance in the genesis of vegetations which comprise a heterogeneous deposit of platelets, fibrin, bacteria and a few inflammatory cells.

Lesions tend to form around the site of maximal velocity blood flow, e.g. on the ventricular surface of the aortic valve and the atrial surface of the mitral. Satellite lesions may form where the regurgitant jet strikes the chordae in aortic incompetence and the left atrial wall in mitral incompetence.

It is postulated that sterile fibrin platelet vegetations pre-exist in circumstances of turbulent flow which are colonized during bacteraemia.

Vegetation morphology and friability, and therefore the embolic potential, varies with the nature of the organism. Heavy bacterial colonization in the protected environment of the avascular fibrin mesh leads to almost continuous bacteraemia. With effective antibiotic treatment vegetations may heal with fibrosis and resultant valve deformity.

Clinical manifestations

Symptoms usually appear within 2 weeks of infection. Nevertheless, IE can present in many ways, which can be considered under the following broad categories:

1. Local tissue destruction. Leaflet perforation, chordal destruction, valve-ring and myocardial abscesses have drastic haemodynamic consequences. Heart block, pyopericardium, aneurysms at the sinuses of Valsalva and intracardiac fistulae may occur.

2. Microscopic and macroscopic embolization. Half of autopsied subjects have evidence of coronary embolization which is usually clinically silent. Left heart vegetations embolize systemically especially to areas of high blood flow. Pulmonary embolism arises from right heart and left to right shunt endocarditis. Septic emboli can produce mycotic aneurysms which may rupture years after bacteriological cure.

3. Immune system activation. Glomerulonephritis (usually focal), arthritis, vasculitis, splenomegaly, and Osler's subcutaneous nodes are results of considerable stimulation of the immune system through persistent antigenaemia.

4. Systemic features. The usual scenario is a patient with prolonged pyrexia and a murmur who has had blood cultures. IE is highly likely if:

- Bacteraemia is sustained (i.e. present in >2 cultures 1 hour apart)
- Typical organisms (e.g. viridans streptococci) are isolated especially in the absence of peripheral phlebitis or indwelling intravascular catheters.

5. Fever. Usually low-grade (<38°C) and spiking, fever is almost universal except in elderly and severely debilitated patients or with congestive failure. Chills occur with acute IE or salicylate treatment.

6. Murmurs are present in 99% of symptomatic patients except in some acute or right-sided IE. The appearance of a new or changed murmur is, however, relatively uncommon and usually reflects acute IE or developing CCF. It is nevertheless important to consider IE in any fever of >1 week associated with a heart murmur.

7. Splinter haemorrhages (sub-ungual dark red striae) are more suggestive if they occur in the proximal nailbed. Toes may be involved. Splinters are more likely to reflect coincidental trauma than IE. *Roth* spots are retinal haemorrhages often oval and pale centred usually near the optical disc and occur in <5% patients with IE. They may also occur in other vasculitides.

8. Splenomegaly (sometimes with infarction) and petechiae each occur in a third of patients. Petechiae are more usually due to vasculitis.

9. Finger–toe clubbing generally occurs only in prolonged disease. Tender small Osler's nodes occur in 10–25% cases on fingers, toe pads, soles, forearms and ears: they may become necrotic. Nontender 1–4 mm haemorrhagic macular areas in palms and soles (called Janeway lesions) may be due to septic emboli.

10. Neurological manifestations include embolization especially to the middle cerebral artery territory. Mycotic aneurysms and brain abscesses purulent meningitis, cranial nerve palsy and cerebral arteritis may occur. Unusually severe localized headaches may suggest a mycotic aneurysm.

11. Congestive heart failure is the most common complication and results from a combination of valve destruction, myocarditis, coronary emboli, myocardial abscesses enhanced by systemic toxaemia and anaemia.

12. Renal insufficiency may result from renal hypoperfusion and vasculitis.

13. Differential diagnosis. IE-like syndromes may be seen in vasculitides, SLE, atrial myxomas, sickle crises and acute rheumatic activity.

Microbiological diagnosis First blood cultures are positive in >95% of patients and bacteraemia is usually continous (98% chance of a culture 1 hour later being positive). Bacterial concentrations are usually low (<100 bacteria per ml blood). Arterial blood offers no advantage over venous. Three cultures are recommended with careful skin preparation and stringent aseptic techniques. At least 10 ml blood should be sampled. It should be diluted 10-fold in both anaerobic and aerobic media.

Negative cultures occur in 25% of antibiotic-treated cases but may also be due to fastiduous organisms like *Brucella*, *Chlamydia*, *Coxiella* (Q fever) *Aspergillus* or *Histoplasma*. 'Recovery' of positive cultures may take up to 2 weeks but usually occurs within 2–3 days.

Treatment

Antibiotics and surgery have had a dramatic impact on what was previously a sure killer. High concentrations of bactericidal antibiotics given for prolonged periods (minimum 2 weeks) are essential to attack the high densities of bacteria protected from host defences and in a state of reduced metabolic activity.

Therapy should be initiated as soon as possible but where diagnostic uncertainty exists it is better to start treatment e.g. amoxycillin and gentamycin after obtaining all microbiological samples.

Treatment should be determined after close consultation with the microbiologist.

1. Initial therapy. Until culture/sensitivity results become available therapy is guided by clinical characteristics. Intracardiac prosthesis-related IE is usually due to *S. aureus* and *S. epidermidis* often methicillin-resistant, and sometimes Gram-negative rods. Therapy should therefore include vancomycin. The same organisms are usually causative in intravenous drug abusers. In subacute situations initial therapy should cover the most 'difficult' potential pathogen (enterococcus).

2. Subsequent therapy. Is guided by the available antibiotic sensitivity results and the least toxic regimen chosen. Therapy should be parenteral and should be effective throughout the 24 hour period. At least 2 weeks treatment is essential. Home or oral therapy can only be allowed after 2 weeks for quick responding cases with haemodynamically uncomplicated IE and an organism sensitive to Penicillin.

Response usually occurs within 3–7 days of antibiotic initiation. Weight gain and return of appetite, resolution of Osler's nodes and splenomegaly may take several weeks.

Persistence/recurrence of pyrexia may indicate a myocardial or metastatic abscess, superinfection or antibiotic fever. Positive blood cultures after several days of treatment indicate an infection or abscess or staphylococcal, enterococcal IE.

Relapse

The majority of relapses occur within 4 weeks of stopping treatment. It is usual to repeat blood cultures 2–4 weeks after stopping antibiotics.

Re-infection

Occurs in 6%.

Surgery

Is required if valve dysfunction is producing CCF. It is dangerous to wait for 'sterilization' of the septic focus because CCF has a tendency to worsen with a serious increase in surgical risks. Leaking aortic valves producing CCF are especially dangerous.

Surgery is also required if medical therapy fails to produce appropriate clinical or bacteriological response. Tricuspid valve endocarditis is often treated with surgery in the first instance because of the high risk of further infection in the event of the addict returning to intravenous drug abuse. Many surgeons are reluctant to insert a tricuspid valve prosthesis in an intravenous drug abuser who has had tricuspid valve endocarditis, due to the likelihood for re-infection, following further drug abuse. Such patients may simply have the tricuspid valve (and any associated infection) resected and high dose antibiotics continued as treatment.

Prophylaxis

Patients with high risk anatomy must be made aware of their condition with optimization of oral health. Antibiotic cover is recommended for certain procedures but there is still some debate about the efficacy and necessity of such measures (refer to regularly updated guidelines e.g. in British National Formulary).

1. High risk anatomy

- Prosthetic valves (both metal and tissue).
- Previous IE.
- Most congenital malformations, except isolated secundum ASD.
- Rheumatic and other acquired valve lesions.
- Hypertrophic obstructive cardiomyopathy.
- Mitral prolapse with incompetence.

2. High bacteraemia-risk procedures

- Oral or pharyngeal procedures inducing mucosal bleeding (dental, tonsillectomy, etc.).
- Surgery affecting intestinal, respiratory or infected urinary mucosa.
- Rigid but not fibreoptic bronchoscopy.
- Oesophageal dilatation/varix injection.
- Excision/drainage of infected tissue.
- Vaginal delivery in the presence of infection.
- Vaginal hysterectomy.

3. Generally not requiring antibiotic cover

- Cardiac catheterization.
- Fibreoptic gastrointestinal (GI) endoscopy/ biopsy.
- Uncomplicated urethral catheterization.
- Uncomplicated vaginal delivery.

Further reading

Acar J, Michel PL, Varenne O, Michaud P, Rafik T. Surgical treatment of infective endocarditis. [Review]. *European Heart Journal*, 1995; **16** Suppl B: 80–3.

Besnier JM, Choutet P. Medical treatment of infective endocarditis. General principles [Review]. *European Heart Journal*, 1995; **16** Suppl B: 80–3. Hogevik H, Olaison L, Andersson R, Lindberg J,. Alestig K. Epidemiological aspects of infective endocarditis in an urban population. A 5 year prospective study [Review]. *Medicine*, 1995; **74**(6): 324–39.

Mathew J, Addai T, Anand A, Morrobel A, Maheshwari P, Freels S. Clinical features, site of involvement, bacteriologic findings, and outcome of infective endocarditis in intravenous drug users. *Archives of Internal Medicine*, 1995; **155**(15): 1641–8.

Prevention of bacterial endocarditis. Recommendations of the American Heart Association. *Journal of the American Medical Association*, 1997; **277:** 1794–801.

ISCHAEMIC HEART DISEASE – ANGINA

Definition

This is a sensation of chest pain when myocardial ischaemia develops secondary to inadequate perfusion to the myocardium and/or when oxygen demands exceeds supply. Metabolic changes, including cellular acidosis and lactate release occur before ST segment depression on the ECG, which in turn preceeds the symptoms of angina.

Classification

1. Stable angina.
2. Unstable angina.
3. Prinzmetal or variant angina.

Stable angina. Typical angina presents as chest tightness or heaviness occurring on exertion and relieved by rest. Angina is typically made worse by exercise, heavy meals, cold weather and emotional stress. Other important precipitating cardiac factors are anaemia, uncontrolled hypertension, left ventricular outflow tract obstruction (aortic valve stenosis, hypertrophic cardiomyopathy), paroxysmal tachyarrhythmias, etc. In stable angina, there is no history to suggest an increase in severity or frequency and angina attacks are usually predictable in nature. There may or may not be ST segment depression on the ECG.

Occasionally angina can be induced by lying down at night or during sleep, which is often referred to as 'decubitus' or nocturnal angina. This is related to an increase in the left ventricular end diastolic volume and hence left ventricular wall stress on lying flat. It may respond to a diuretic, nitrate or calcium antagonist taken in the evening.

Unstable angina. This usually refers to angina of increasing frequency and severity which is induced by increasingly minimum effort or coming on at rest. However many definitions of unstable angina exist. The underlying pathophysiology is thrombus overlying a ruptured atherosclerotic plaque.

The usual accepted definitions include angina occurring with increasing frequency or severity, or angina occurring at rest or with increasing minimal exertion. Fresh symptoms are often associated with ST depression on the ECG and symptoms are relieved less easily with GTN sprays or tablets. If untreated, this has a high rate of progression onto mycardial infarction and this should be regarded as a pre-infarction situation. True unstable angina therefore represents an acute medical emergency.

Variant angina. This is angina occurring associated with transient ST segment elevation on the ECG. This is associated with coronary artery spasm, with or without additional arteriosclerotic lesions. There is prompt relief of ST segment elevation by nitrates or calcium antagonists. The condition is unusual, and may very rarely progress on to cause myocardial infarction.

Silent mycardial ischaemia. Silent mycardial ischaemia occurs when episodes of ST depression on the ECG occur without chest pain and can be documented on an exercise test or during 24 h Holter monitoring. Silent, asymptomatic ST depression has been found to be present in 2.5% of the male population, and may be more common in diabetics, especially if autonomic neuropathy is present.

Silent mycardial ischaemia is commonly seen in patients with chronic stable angina, where up to 75% of episodes of ST depression on 24 h Holter monitor may be silent. Silent ischaemia is more commonly seen in the morning and is mirrored by the increased incidents of myocardial infarction in the early hours of the morning. The evidence suggests that silent ischaemia has the same prognostic implications as symptomatic angina and thus, such patients should be investigated along conventional lines with exercise testing and coronary angiography if necessary.

Management of angina

This requires application of non-pharmacologal measures, that include alteration of lifestyle, exclusion or treatment of precipitating factors; and drug treatment, with possibly progression on to invasive cardiac investigation, and revascularization with surgery or angioplasty.

Non-pharmacological measures include lifestyle alterations, that may require reduction of physical activity at work or at home. Weight reduction may be necessary and a change of diet (especially if co-existent hypercholesterolaemia is present) may be necessary. Smoking should be stopped.

Precipitating factors for angina, such as anaemia, thyroid disease, high output states, diabetes and hypercholesterolaemia should be indentified and treated. Twenty-four hour Holter ECG monitoring should be performed if the history suggests arrhythmias precipitating angina.

Exercise testing is performed on patients with stable angina and helps confirm the diagnosis, assess the severity of symptoms and exercise capacity, and is a suitable guide to the need for coronary angiography.

If patients cannot undertake exercise treadmill testing, another option is pharmocological stress testing using myocardial perfusion scanning, which uses a pharmacological stressor (such as dipyridamole or adenosine) and a radionuclide substance (thallium). The radioisotope identifies either fixed perfusion defects (previous mycardial infarction) or reversible defects (defects seen on stress or exertion, which redistributes during rest).

Medical management

Drug therapy of angina involves three classes of drugs. There are the nitrates, beta blockers and calcuim antagonists. Recently a new class of anti-anginal drugs has been introduced, that is the potassium channel openers. Unstable angina requires additional treatment with anti-thrombotic therapy.

Stable angina is initially treated with aspirin and a short-acting nitrate to be used sublingually as required. If symptoms get worse a beta blocker should be introduced, but if these are contra-indicated (for example in severe peripheral vascular disease, bronchospasm, low output states, left ventricular failure, Prinzmetals variant angina, heart block, Raynaud's phenomenon) then calcium antagonists are the drugs of choice. There is some evidence that verapamil and diltizem may have benefits in this situation, but the evidence suggests that short acting calcium antagonists, especially those from the dihydropyridine group (for example nifedipine) may have an adverse effect. Nevertheless most calcium antagonists now come in long acting preparations but current guidelines suggest the use of a dihydropyridine together with a beta blocker to avoid the cathecholamine surges associated with dihydropyridine calcium antagnonists.

Further uncontrolled stable angina despite aspirin, beta blocker and sublingual nitrate will require the addition of a calcium antagonist and/or an oral nitrate preparation. Potassium channel openers have recently been introduced and are licenced as first line drugs for angina. As there is little outcome data from this class of drugs, our clinical practice is to use these drugs as second or third line therapy in addition to other established treatments.

Management of unstable angina involves the use of anti-anginal drugs as outlined above. Patients also require treatment with anti-thrombotic therapy including aspirin and heparin, and patients who do not settle on medical treatment require urgent invasive investigation with cardiac catherization.

Initial managment of unstable angina requires bed rest, light sedation and analgesia as required. Triple therapy with established anti-anginal drugs such as beta blocker, nitrate and calcium antagonists should be instituted, and aspirin should be started. Aspirin has in fact been shown to reduce the incidence of myocardial infarction and mortality in unstable angina. There is also evidence that anti-coagulation with intravenous heparin helps with unstable angina and that the benefits of heparin may be additive to those of aspirin.

New developments in antithrombotic therapy in unstable angina include the glycoprotein IIb IIIa inhibitor class of drugs.

Thrombolytic therapy (for example, streptokinase) has been found to be of no benefit in unstable angina. Beta blockers should be avoided if there is any suggestion that the unstable angina is due to coronary spasm. It should also be noted that calcium antagonists have not been shown to reduce mortality in unstable angina when used alone but may increase the incidence of myocardial infarction and recurrent unstable symptoms; nevertheless, they are generally safe and useful when used as additive treatment to a beta blocker.

If symptoms of unstable angina are not settling despite the treatment regime suggested above, intravenous nitrates should be added. Coronary angiography will be required when symptoms have settled, but more urgently if pain continues. Recent evidence suggests that an aggressive intervention policy is associated with more morbidity and mortality, and patients should therefore be stablized and settled before intervention, if possible. Approxmately 10% of patients have left main coronary artery stenosis and about 70% with left anterior descending artery stenosis. However, <3% of patients have coronary spasms and <10% have normal coronary arteries.

ISCHAEMIC HEART DISEASE – MYOCARDIAL INFARCTION

Significant hypoxia of myocardium as a result of cardiac ischaemia leads to myocardial infarction. Approximately 95% of patients with myocardial infarction have total occlusion of the relevant coronary artery within 4 h of pain onset. The majority of occlusions are associated with intimal plaque rupture and haemorrhage into the plaque. The minority of patients will have normal coronary arteries and emboli or spasm are the mechanisms in these cases.

The mortality of myocardial infarctions if untreated is approximately 40% in the first 4 weeks and 50% of these patients die within the first 2 h of symptoms. Hospital mortality has dramatically reduced in the last few years and is approximately 10%. The primary problem therefore is to avoid delay in getting heart attack patients to hospital and initiation of established therapy, such as thrombolysis – leading to establishment of ideal 'door-to-needle' times for initiation of thrombolysis and the realization that 'minutes is myocardium', as further delays before treatment and revascularization leads to graeter myocardial ischaemia and damage.

Education of lay people in cardiac resusitation as well as the development of mobile coronary care units are important advances, allowing the the reduction of deaths during transport from home to hospital, improved resuscitation of cardiac arrests, early treatment of cardiac arrhythmias, early administration of thrombolysis and reduction of time taken to reach a hospital coronary care unit.

Diagnosis

The diagnosis is based on typical history, ECG changes and cardiac enzyme elevation by twofold. Other findings which may be present include physical signs (for example pericardial rub, dyskinetic cardiac apex), a mild pyrexia developing 48 h after the pain.

Cardiac enzyme changes are usually detected by measurement of creatine phosphate kinase and its MB isoenzyme. This is the most specific cardiac enzyme and rises and falls within the first 72 h of a heart attack. Peak concentrations occur 24 h post-infarction and enzymes start to rise after 6 h.

Other measured enzymes include aspartate transaminase (AST) which is less specific than CPK–MB and rises and falls within 4–6 days. The peak concentration is again at 24 h. However, AST is also elevated in liver disease and hepatic congestion, pulmonary embolism, muscle injury, shock or intramuscular injection.

Late rise in cardiac enzymes can be detected by measurement of lactic dehydrogenase (LDH) which is again not cardiac specific. The peak rise occurs at 4–5 days post-infarction and may take 2 weeks to return to base line. Abnormal LDH can also be seen in haemolysis, leukaemia, renal disease, etc.

Other markers of myocardial injury such as myoglobin (peak <6 h) and troponin T (specific for mycardial infarction and are raised up to 2 weeks following infarction) have been suggested.

Management

Patients with suspected myocardial infarction should have a fast track system to the coronary care unit. Immediate assessment should include examination for the presence of shock, heart failure, hypotension or new murmurs; this should be followed by establishment of IV access, and a 12 lead ECG.

Initial treatment should be oral aspirin 150 mg od, and oxygen. Analgesia such as diamorphine should be given to control pain, as well as sublingual nitrate. Thrombolysis should be started as soon as possible and additional therapy such as beta blockers, nitrates, heparin and ACE inhibitors should be considered.

Thrombolytic therapy is usually with streptokinase 1.5 M units intravenously, and the effect is additive to aspirin (ISIS-2). Streptokinase is antigenic, and administration is associated with allergic reactions and hypotension; its use also generates antibodies, which may neutralize subsequent administration. In patients who have previously received streptokinase, recombinant tissue plasminogen activator (rtPA) 100 mg is used if thrombolysis is needed again. rtPA has also been advocated in hypotensive patients, and in young patients with anterior myocardial infarction, in view of the greater patency rates and marginal mortality advantage over streptokinase (GUSTO). All thrombolytic agents may cause bleeding, including strokes, and the antagonist (if needed) is tranexamic acid.

Beta-blocking agents have been shown to reduce mortality and subsequent cardiac events. Early mortality is reduced by preventing cardiac rupture

(ISIS-1), late mortality is by preventing recurrent infarction, but these drugs are contraindicated in pulmonary oedema, peripheral ischaemia and brochospasm.

The use of routine heparin is controversial. Low dose (5000 IU b.d. or t.i.d.) subcutaneous heparin prevents deep venous thrombosis and high dose (12500 IU b.d.) subcutaneous heparin prevents mural thrombus especially in anterior myocardial infarction. Heparin does add to the thrombolytic effects of tissue plasminogen activator and intravenous heparin should therefore be continued for 24 h to improve coronary patency.

The routine use of IV or oral nitrates should be confined to those with left ventricular failure or continuing angina. There is little evidence that routine administration of nitrates alters mortality (ISIS-4). Recently the use of ACE inhibitors post-myocardial infarction, especially in patients with evidence of left ventricular dysfunction has reduced long-term mortality and morbidity (recurrent heart failure and reinfarction). These drugs are effective in reducing left ventricular dilatation, with beneficial effects on left ventricular remodeling.

Patients particularly with large infarcts, clinical evidence of heart failure, cardiomegaly on the chest X-ray, anterior lead T-waves on the ECG or left ventricular ejection fraction <40% on echocardiography or nuclear scanning, would particularly benefit from ACE inhibitors (up to 60 lives saved per 1000). By contrast, prescription of ACE inhibitors to every heart attack patient, irrespective of cardiac function, would only confer a modest mortality benefit (4 per 1000, from ISIS-4).

Routine use of IV magnesium is controversial, with evidence from the LIMIT-2 study suggesting that a reduction in mortality by 24%, whilst data from the larger ISIS-4 study refutes this, suggesting that magnesium may even be detelerious, with a slight excess in mortality.

Calcium antagonists may be used in selected patients; for example diltiazem may be used in non-Q myocardial infarction (MDPIT study), whilst verapamil may be used through post-myocardial infarction but only if left ventricular function is not impaired (DAVITT-2).

Primary PTCA without thrombolysis has recently been advocated as being successful in reducing reinfarction, death and intracranial bleeding, when compared to conventional thrombolytic therapy. Myocardial salvage is similar with either technique. However, use of primary PTCA as the initial treatment for myocardial infarction requires considerable logistic support and specialist centres.

Post-myocardial infarction management

This should include cardiovascular risk factor assessment and early investigation for other high risk features such as left ventricular dysfunction or underlying remaining cardiac ischaemia.

There is also evidence to recommend the use of soluble aspirin, 150 mg od, and a routine beta blocker, both of which have been independently shown to reduce subsequent recurrent cardiac events. For example, the evidence suggests a reduction in mortality by 20% and reinfarction by 33% in patients taking aspirin.

Beta blockers should be continued for a least 2 years and possibly 5 years post-infarction, and aspirin indefinitely. ACE inhibitors in patients with left ventricular dysfunction has also been validated as established treatment. The use of aggressive lipid lowering strategies, including lipid lowering agents such as the statins, have been shown to reduce long-term mortality and morbidity (4S, CARE studies). Long-term calcium antagonists are, however, of doubtful value.

Patients with high risk post-myocardial infarction are those with unstable angina, ventricular arrhythmias, cardiomegaly on the chest X-ray, poor left ventricular function on echocardiography on nuclear scanning (left ventricular ejection fraction <40%), a positive exercise treadmill testing at stage II or less on the Bruce protocol and those with frequent episodes of silent ischaemia on 24 h Holter monitoring. Such patients should be considered for early invasive investigation and possible revascularization procedures.

Further reading

4S Study Group. Randomised trial of cholesterol lowering in 4444 patients with coronary heart disease: the Scandinavian Simvastatin Survival Study. *Lancet*, 1994; **344:** 1383–89.

Furberg CD, Psaty BM, Meyer JV. Nifedipine dose-related increase in mortality in patients with coronary heart disease. *Circulation*, 1995; **92:** 1326–31.

Grines CL, Browne KF, Marco J *et al.* Primary angioplasty in myocardial infarction study group. A comparison of immediate angioplasty with thrombolytic therapy for acute myocardial infarction. *New England Journal of Medicine,* 1993; **328:** 673–79.

Hansen JF. Effect of verapamil on mortality and major events after acute myocardial infarction. The Danish Verapamil Infarction Trial II – DAVITT II. *American Journal of Cardiology,* 1990; **66:** 779–85.

Ryan TJ, Faxon DP, Gunnar RM *et al.* Guidelines for percutaneous transluminal coronary angioplasty: a report of the American College of Cardiology/American Heart Association Task Force on assessment of diagnostic and therapeutic cardiovascular procedures. *Journal American College of Cardiologists,* 1988; **12:** 529–45.

Sacks RM, Pfeffer MA, Moye L *et al.* The effect of pravastatin on coronary events after myocardial infarction in patients with average cholesterol levels. *New England Journal of Medicine,* 1996; **335:** 1001–9.

LIPIDS AND HEART DISEASE

The total serum cholesterol is a strong predictor of coronary artery disease and reduction of serum cholesterol, particularly in patients with very high levels, reduces cardiovascular risk. There is now significant evidence that reduction in serum cholesterol is important in the prevention of ischaemic heart disease.

Classification of lipids

Lipoproteins are usually characterized according to their density and their appearance on electrophoretic assays. These consist of chylomicrons, very low density lipoproteins (VLDL), intermediate density lipoproteins (IDL), low density lipoproteins (LDL) and high density lipoproteins (HDL).

Apoproteins are the protective components of lipoproteins. Apo A is synthesized by both the intestine and the liver and is the main component of HDL. Apo B has two main types: apo B_{48} is produced in the intestine and only found in chylomicrons while apo B_{100} is found in chylomicrons, VLDL and LDL. Apo C is a major constituent of VLDL and apo E is transported as a constituent of chylomicrons, VLDL, IDL and HDL.

1. Lipoprotein function. Chylomicrons are responsible for transporting dietary triglyceride (90% of their mass) from the intestine and into the circulation while LDL transport 75% of the total plasma cholesterol. HDL are synthesized in the liver and intestine and have a major role in the mobilization of tissue cholesterol. VLDL are synthesized in the liver and intestine and their main function is to transport triglyceride.

Lipoprotein (a) or Lp(a) consists of one LDL particle and one molecule of apolipoprotein (a), and is a molecule associated with thrombogenesis and atherogenesis.

2. Lipids and ischaemic disease. Several prospective epidemiological studies have demonstrated that raised levels of LDL-cholesterol and low levels of HDL-cholesterol are independent risk factors for ischaemic heart disease. In addition, a number of clinical and population studies have linked elevated triglyceride levels and increased plasma levels of Lp(a) to the presence, extent and progression of atherosclerosis.

The long-term outcome of atheroma regression studies have demonstrated beneficial clinical and angiographic effects. More recently, a number of large-scale studies have addressed the role of lipid lowering in terms of primary and secondary prevention of coronary events.

Atheroma regression trials *Program on the Surgical Control of Hyperlipidaemias (POSCH) study.* This trial used regional ileal bypass surgery to reduce cholesterol levels in patients with a history of coronary artery disease and total cholesterol level above 5.7 mmol/l or LDL-cholesterol above 3.6 mmol/l. The long-term follow-up demonstrated clear angiographic and clinical benefits. Several shorter regression studies using hydroxy-methylglutaryl (HMG) co-A reductase inhibitors (statins) support the results of the POSCH trial.

Secondary prevention trials There have been numerous intervention trials which have studied the effect of cholesterol reduction, with diet and drugs, in patients with coronary heart disease. Most of these trials had low statistical power and failed to demonstrate convincing benefit from lipid lowering. However, two recent large-scale intervention trials, using the more powerful statin drugs, have demonstrated clear benefits.

1. Scandanavian Simvastatin Survival (SSSS) Study. This placebo-controlled trial studied the effects of cholesterol reduction in 4444 patients with total cholesterol levels between 5.5 and 8.0 mmol/l and a history of angina pectoris or previous MI. Simvastatin reduced total cholesterol by 25%, LDL-cholesterol by 35% and increased HDL-cholesterol by 8%. In the treatment group the results were significant with a 30% reduction in all cause mortality, a 42% risk reduction in deaths from ischaemic heart disease, a 34% reduction in cardiovascular mortality and a 37% risk reduction in coronary revascularization procedures.

2. Cholesterol and Recurrent Events (CARE) Study. This double-blind placebo-controlled trial aimed to study the effects of cholesterol reduction with pravastatin, in patients with a previous history of MI and a total cholesterol level below 6.2 mmol/l. The LDL-cholesterol had to be within the range 3.0–4.5 mmol/l, triglycerides below 4.0 mmol/l. Pravastatin significantly reduced the risk of coronary death or non-fatal recurrent MI by 24%, reduced the total risk of MI (fatal or non-fatal) by 25%, with a 27% reduction in the requirement for coronary revascularization procedures.

Primary prevention trials
A number of primary prevention trials have failed to demonstrate convincing benefit from cholesterol reduction in those patients without a previous history of ischaemic heart disease. These include the Los Angeles Veterans Diet Trial, the WHO Clofibrate trial, the Helsinki Heart trial (using gemfibrozil) and the Lipid Research Clinics cholestyramine trial.

However, the first long-term primary prevention study using a statin drug, the West of Scotland Coronary Prevention Study (WOSCOPS), demonstrated benefits in high risk men most without a history of ischaemic heart disease. A total of 6595 men with LDL-cholesterol levels above 4.0 mmol/l at two screening visits, or between 4.5 and 6.0 mmol/l at one visit, were randomized to receive pravastatin, 40 mg daily or placebo. The men were followed-up for a mean period of 4.9 years.

Pravastatin significantly reduced the risk of coronary heart disease death by 28%, with a 22% reduction in overall mortality and a 37% reduction in coronary revascularization procedures.

Management of hyperlipidaemia
The majority of patients should receive an adequate trial of dietary modification before lipid lowering drug therapy is considered. In addition the secondary causes of dyslipidaemia should be addressed, including hypothyroidism, diabetes, chronic renal disease and high alcohol intake.

1. Secondary prevention. Lipid-lowering drug therapy should be considered in all patients with persistent hyperlipidaemia and a history of coronary artery disease. Statin therapy should be considered for patients with a history of MI and a total cholesterol greater than 4.8 mmol/l (or LDL > 3.2 mmol/l), or those who have angina pectoris and total cholesterol above 5.2 mmol/l. Lipid-lowering therapy should also be considered in patients with persistent hyperlipidaemia who have undergone coronary artery bypass grafting or coronary angioplasty.

2. Primary prevention. There is a role for lipid-lowering therapy in the treatment of men without clinically apparent vascular disease but who, nevertheless, have a high risk of developing overt coronary heart disease. This includes patients with multiple coronary risk factors and a total cholesterol above 5.5 mmol/l (or LDL >3.7 mmol/l).

Further reading

Buchwald H, Varco RL, Matts JP, *et al.* Effect of partial ileal bypass on mortality and morbidity from coronary heart disease in patients with hypercholesterolaemia: report of the Program on the Surgical Control of Hyperlipidaemias (POSCH). *New England Journal of Medicine,* 1990; **323:** 946–55.

Sachs FM, Pfeffer MA, Moye LA, *et al.* The effect of pravastatin on coronary events after myocardial infarction in patients with average cholesterol levels. *New England Journal of Medicine,* 1996; **335:** 1001–9.

Shepherd J, Cobbe M, Ford I, *et al.* for the West of Scotland Coronary Prevention Study Group. Prevention of coronary heart disease with pravastatin in men with hypercholesterolaemia. *New England Journal of Medicine,* 1995; **333:** 1301–7.

The Scandanavian Simvastatin Survival Group. Randomised trial of cholesterol lowering in 444 patients with coronary heart disease. The Scandanavian Simvastatin Survival Study (4S) *Lancet,* 1994; **344:** 1383.

PACEMAKERS

Indications for temporary pacing

1. Sinus bradycardia or arrest; if not responding to atropine in the symptomatic patient.

2. Gen eral anaesthesia; or postoperatively, in the same circumstances as above.

3. Drug overdose, if the patient is symptomatic and not responding to supportive measures.

4. AV block in acute MI

- Complete heart block - if inferior MI, this is often transient and responds to atropine.
- Mobitz type II block.
- Trifasicular block as in alternating Lt and Rt bundle branch block (BBB).
- (Debatable) when the P-R interval is prologed in the presence of either new LtBBBor new RtBBB with left anterior or posterior hemiblock.

5. Other indications include cardiac surgery adjacent to the AVNode or other parts of the cardiac conduction system. Overdrive pacing can be used for tachyarrhythmias not responding to usual antiarrhythmic treatment and requiring (or intolerant of) frequent cardioversion.

Indications for permanent pacing

1. Sick sinus syndrome or sinus node disease; only when symptomatic, where the patient should receive a permanent atrial pacemaker or a dual chamber system if associated with atrioventricular nodal disease (as in 30% of the cases).

2. Atrioventricular nodal disease

- Acquired CHB.
- Congenital CHB: under the circumstances mentioned elsewhere in the section on bradyarrhythmias.
- Mobitz type II AV block.
- Trifasicular block as mentioned above.

Pacing and other devices for tachyarrhythmias

Recently a variety of programmable pacemaker devices has been developed to treat some tachyarrhythmias. They can be programmed for overdrive or underdrive pacing, or by delivering bursts of extrastimuli. Antitachycardia devices are usually used when drug treatment is unsatisfactory or results in serious side-effects, as well as in patients with poor LV function or in female patients wishing to become pregnant (in whom antiarrhythmic drugs are contraindicated).

Using the same principle, the implantable cardioverter defibrillator (IVCD) for malignant ventricular arrhythmias (ventricular tachycardia and ventricular fibrillation) and the atrial defibrillator device (for paroxysmal atrial fibrillation) are recent developments for managing resistant tachyarrhythmias.

After atrioventricular node ablation or modification (using high energy radiofrequency waves) for elective rate control in fast atrial fibrillation unresponsive to drugs, permanent pacemaker implantation may also be needed.

Other indications for permanet pacemakers include patients with hypertrophic obsructive cardiomyopathy with persistent symptoms, such as syncope or near syncope episodes, as well as limiting dyspnoea, might benefit from a permanent dual chamber pacemaker system with special programming to shorten the atrioventricular delay and pre-excite the ventricles. This may improve filling and reduce outflow tract gradient. Patients with cartoid sinus hypersensitivity syndrome also require dual chamber pacing

Pacemaker code and nomenclature

In 1974 Parsonnet introduced the three letter code, which is currently used with some modifications. The first letter refers to the paced chamber, the second to the sensed one and the third to the response to the sensed impulse; either triggered or inhibited. A fourth letter indicates whether the pacemaker is rate-responsive; a fifth letter if the pacemaker is programmable or not; and a sixth letter if telemetric facilities are provided. For example, a DDDR pacemaker signifies that both ('dual') right atrium and ventricle are paced and sensed, and the response is both triggered or inhibited (the third letter being 'D' for 'dual'); the 'R' indicates the system is rate responsive.

Pacing modalities

1. Unipolar systems. Most permanent units are unipolar, deploying the box as the anode and the wire as a cathode. The pacing spike is large when detected on the surface ECG.

2. Bipolar systems. This is similar to most temporary pacing leads. It results in a smaller pacing spike and may be used routinely or if the patient is particularly at risk of external interference by electromyographic inhibiton, faulty electric motors and vibration.

3. Single chamber pacing. For example, a single right atrial pacemaker lead (AAI system) is required for sinus node disease, unless associated with atrioventricular conduction block. The latter should be tested for, either before the implantation or by pacing the atrium at fast heart rates after the implantation of the atrial lead, to check for evidence of atrioventricular conduction block, for example, Weinkebac block at heart rate of above 110–120/min.

VVI pacing may be used for ventricular pacing especially if the patient is in slow AF or has low level of mobility or concomitant medical problems.

4. Dual chamber pacing is considered by many to be the ideal pacing mode for patients with CHB as it achieves physiological pacing, where the ventricular pacing rate increases in response to exercise and maintains AV synchrony. Other advantages are that the risk of AF may be reduced (compared to VVI pacing) and pacemaker syndrome is avoided. The latter occurs whereby the patient develops symptoms due to absence of atrioventricular synchrony. Atrial contraction against a closed A-V valve may give rise to palpitations; reduced ventricular filling may cause hypotension and dizziness.

Complications of pacemaker wire insertion

1. Pneumothorax. A chest X-ray should be done post-implantation to check the wire position and to rule out pneumothorax or haemothorax.

2. Infection. This is a catastropic complication often necessitating removal of the entire pacemaker system and reimplantation at another site.

3. Thrombophlebitis. This rarely occurs in the subclavian or cephalic vein, but is more likely if several wires have been deployed and long-term warfarin may be necessary.

4. Arrhythmias. Atrial leads may result in atrial tachyarrhythmias and the ventricular lead can cause ventricular arrhythmias during manipulation at implantation.

General advice

The patients should be warned that the unipolar system may rarely be inhibited by powerful alternating electromagnetic fields. Ionizing radiation can damage the unit and it may be necessary to to shield the pacemaker. Magnetic fields (such as magnetic resonance imaging scanning) should be avoided.

Diathermy should be as far away as possible from the pacemaker, and any suspected inhibition by being too near the diathermy electrode can be overcome by placing a magnet over the unit to convert it to VOO mode which then paces continuously at a fixed rate. Resuscitation equipment should be made available.

The patient with a permanent pacemaker can hold an ordinary driving licence, but not a HGV or PSV licence. They can drive after 1 month of implantation and they do not need to pay any special insurance.

Further reading

Moses HW *et al. A Practical Guide to Cardiac Pacing.* Boston: Little Brown & Co., 3rd Edn, 1991.

Related topic of interest

Arrhythmias – bradyarrhythmias (p. 34)

PERIPHERAL VASCULAR DISEASE

Peripheral vascular disease (PVD) is very common, the symptoms affecting approximately 10% of the population over 70 years of age. The cause in the overwhelming majority is atherosclerosis but rarer causes of peripheral ischaemia are Buerger's disease, autoimmune vasculitis, inflammatory arteritis (Takayasu's), drugs such as ergotamine, fibromuscular hyperplasia, cystic adventitial degeneration and anatomical entrapment syndromes (popliteal artery entrapment or thoracic outlet syndrome). Risk factors for atherosclerosis are hypertension, diabetes mellitus, cigarette smoking and hyperlipidaemia. Associated ischaemic heart disease and cerebrovascular disease are very common. Abdominal aortic aneurysm co-exists in up to 15% of patients with symptomatic peripheral vascular disease and must be excluded by abdominal ultrasound scan.

Presentation

Early symptoms of PVD are those of intermittent claudication usually affecting the calves. Thigh and buttock pain are indicative of proximal (aortoiliac) disease. Claudication pain occurs only after exercise (e.g. walking – where the claudication distance can be recorded) and is abolished by a few minutes rest. Chronic muscle pain at rest is more likely to be due to myositis and when associated with burning and paraesthesia in the feet, peripheral neuropathy (common in diabetics) or spinal cord compression should be suspected. Intermittent claudication is a relatively benign phenomenon and only 10% of cases eventually progress to critical (limb threatening) ischaemia. As the disease progresses, rest pain in the feet, characteristically worse at night and eased by dependency, may occur followed by ischaemic ulceration and gangrene.

The diagnosis is made clinically from the history together with the findings of absent or reduced pulses and reduction in the ankle brachial pressure index (ABPI). Mild cases may have normal pulses at rest and a normal resting ABPI but the pulses may disappear after exercise with a corresponding fall in the post-exercise ABPI.

Management

All patients with limb-threatening ischaemia should be assessed for some form of revascularization unless the loss of the affected limb would not affect their lifestyle, e.g. the patient being bed bound, paraplegic, previous stroke, etc.; or if their life expectancy is very short due to gross cardiac, pulmonary or malignant disease; or if the affected limb is already beyond salvage due to extensive ischaemic necrosis.

Management of patients with non-disabling claudication involves reassurance and reduction of risk factors (control of hypertension, hyperlipidaemia, diabetes and most importantly cessation of cigarette smoking). Duplex scanning of the peripheral arteries is performed to exclude an abdominal aortic aneurysm and to document the sites and extent of arterial occlusions and stenoses.

1. Drugs. Drugs for the treatment of chronic PVD are largely useless but all patients with symptomatic atherosclerosis should be prescribed aspirin (75–150 mg a day) in the absence of any contraindication. Any reversible medical condition must be treated first especially severe angina, cardiac dysrhythmia, heart failure, uncontrolled diabetes or uncontrolled hypertension in order to minimize any operative risks.

2. Angioplasty. Operative or endovascular intervention is indicated for disabling claudication (especially in those with proximal disease) and strongly indicated for limb-threatening ischaemia.

Percutaneous transluminal angioplasty (PTA) (with or without a stent) may be useful especially in those with localized short segment disease in the iliac or superficial femoral arteries. This allows treatment at a lower risk than with conventional surgery, with a short in-patient stay and often under local anaesthetic. This has allowed definitive treatment to be offered to many claudicants who would hitherto have been treated conservatively. Suitable patients can be identified by high quality duplex scanning. Angiography should be performed for the purposes of planning any operative or endovascular intervention and not for diagnostic purposes. It must be remembered that angiography does have small but definite risks. These are rare but include catheter trauma to the arteries, contrast allergy and renal failure. Many surgeons only recommend treatment of infrainguinal disease if critical ischaemia exists and not for those with claudication. Proximal arterial lesions should be corrected first if possible by PTA.

3. Surgery. Lesions not amenable to PTA can be bypassed using conventional vascular techniques such as aorto-bifemoral grafting or by the extra anatomic route (axillo-femoral or femoro-femoral bypass) in those unfit for a major abdominal procedure. Infra-inguinal disease may be treatable by PTA but usually some form of operative bypass will be necessary. Femoro-distal bypass using autologous vein is now a routine procedure and successful limb salvage can be obtained in up to 80% of patients.

Management in diabetics

The outcome in diabetics is no worse than non-diabetics. Diabetics with tibial artery disease however, pose some exacting technical problems but many have patent vessels at ankle or foot level suitable for reconstructive surgery. Any diabetic with trophic lesions and no palpable foot pulses should be assessed for vascular reconstruction as there may well be a potentially salvageable problem. The ABPI is misleading in these patients due to calcification of the ankle level arteries. Amputation can be avoided in many of these patients, all of whom should be assessed by a vascular surgeon.

Acute arterial insufficiency

This is characterized by the well known 6 'Ps'; Pallor, Pulselessness, Paraesthesiae, Pain, Paralysis, Perishing with cold.

The cause may be arterial thrombosis, embolus, or rarely following a spontaneous aortic dissection. It is often difficult to determine the exact cause clinically. It may arise against a background of claudication indicating a thrombosis. An embolus may occur from the heart in those with recent subendocardial MI, valvular disorders or tachydysrhythmia (including atrial fibrillation), from an ulcerated aortic plaque or from a proximal aortic aneurysm. In any event, early administration of intravenous heparin is indicated. All patients who have sustained an embolus should undergo cardiac assessment to exclude a cardiac source of embolus and also ultrasound examination of the aorta.

If the limb is viable and improving, then there is time to investigate the patient in a relatively leisurely fashion. Many patients will settle on anticoagulation alone. If, however, there is profound ischaemia with motor or sensory deficit then urgent action is required to save the affected limb. Those with severe acute ischaemia whose limbs appear salvageable must be referred immediately to a vascular surgeon. The presence of swollen, indurated tender muscles with fixed lividity of the skin suggests that the situation has gone beyond repair and amputation will need to be considered. However, not infrequently these patients are dying of some other cause and symptomatic treatment only may be appropriate.

Intra-arterial thrombolysis (IAT) with low dose recombitant tissue plasminogen activator (rTPA) is available in most hospitals where vascular surgery is practised and therefore most patients should undergo early angiography. Overall, about 60% of patients with acute arterial insufficiency can be treated successfully with IAT using rTPA. After clot lysis, any underlying atheromatous lesion causing a thrombosis can be treated by PTA or a definitive surgical procedure can be planned. Those in whom IAT is not appropriate or is unsuccessful should proceed to immediate operation. It must be remembered that IAT is not without hazard, the main risks being catheter trauma and haemorrhage either at the puncture site or distant, including retroperitoneal, gastrointestinal or intra-cranial with sometimes fatal results. For this reason many surgeons prefer early operative intervention following angiography.

Carotid artery disease

In patients who have symptomatic internal carotid artery stenosis of >70%, the risks of a subsequent disabling stroke or stroke-related death over the next 3 years is reduced from approximately 25% on medical treatment alone to 7% by carotid endarterectomy. The symptoms which suggest internal carotid artery stenosis are carotid territory transient ischaemic attack (TIA), amaurosis fugax or completed carotid territory non-disabling stroke. Therefore all patients who have sustained a carotid territory event should be evaluated for carotid artery stenosis.

1. Assessment. The presence or absence of a carotid bruit has no predictive value whatsoever in the management of these patients and reliance on this physical sign in order to determine those with significant carotid artery disease should be abandoned forthwith. The use of a 'stroke protocol' to investigate these patients is of great value to ensure precise and appropriate investigation of all relevant systems.

It is important that all these patients undergo cranial CT to determine the precise cerebral pathology and in those with an infarct, carotid duplex scan should be performed. This will detect any carotid artery disease reliably and quantify the degree of stenosis. Investigations of other areas such as the heart, blood pressure, renal function, lipids, serology, autoimmune status, blood sugar and thyroid function should be undertaken. Following investigations, those patients with symptomatic internal carotid artery stenosis >70% will be identified and these should all be referred to a vascular surgeon for consideration of surgery if their general condition allows.

It is most important that the patient is counselled thoroughly as to the risks and benefits of the procedure. Angiography should not be undertaken unless the patient agrees to having an operation performed as this investigation itself carried a 1% risk of stroke in this group of patients and furthermore may not be deemed necessary by all vascular surgeons. Angiography should never be undertaken for purely diagnostic purposes as a first line investigation in patients suspected of having carotid artery disease.

2. Management. Patients being considered for carotid endarterectomy should be referred to a vascular surgeon who regularly undertakes this procedure and has a combined operative mortality and stroke risk of <5%. Otherwise benefits of the procedure are eroded by the operative risks. Whether surgery is to be recommended for asymptomatic stenosis of >70% is debatable. There is some evidence that young (<70 years of age) otherwise fit men do derive protection from ipsilateral stroke by carotid endarterectomy but certainly in the UK this is not widespread practice and the results of future trials are awaited. These patients should be treated with aspirin (75–300 mg daily).

Carotid endarterectomy is not systemically a very stressful procedure for the patient and is well tolerated even by the elderly. Modern methods of intra-operative monitoring using transcranial Doppler scanning of the middle cerebral artery blood flow has been shown to improve operative safety. Postoperatively, patients should be nursed in a high dependency area for 12–24 hours. Operative safety is further improved by attention to risk factors such as hypertension and diabetes preoperatively. Postoperatively patients should be maintained on low dose soluble aspirin.

Follow-up duplex scan of the operated or the contralateral carotid artery in the absence of symptoms should be not undertaken as it has no proven therapeutic benefit and can cause unnecessary anxiety both in the patient and his medical advisors.

Further reading

European Carotid Surgery Trialists' Collaborative Group. European Carotid Surgery Trial: Interim results for symptomatic patients with severe (70–99%) or with mild (0–29%) carotid stenosis. *Lancet*, 1991; **337:** 1235–43.

Executive Committee for the Asymptomatic Carotid Atherosclerosis Study. Endarterectomy for asymptomatic carotid artery stenosis. *JAMA*, 1995; **273:** 1421–8.

North American Symptomatic Carotid Endarterectomy Trial Collaborations. Beneficial effects of carotid endarterectomy in symptomatic patients with high grade stenosis. *New England Journal of Medicine,* 1991; **325:** 445–53.

Related topics of interest

SECONDARY PREVENTION OF HEART DISEASE

Secondary prevention in patients with a history of MI is aimed at reducing the risk of recurrent cardiovascular events and improving mortality. This involves the modification of risk factors and drug therapy.

Risk factor control

1. Smoking. Although there is no direct evidence from randomized trials to confirm the benefits of stopping smoking following a MI, there is clear evidence that smoking promotes atherosclerosis and therefore patients should be strongly encouraged to abstain.

2. Hypertension. There should be strict blood pressure control, with a preference for beta blockers and ACE inhibitors, in order to prevent cardiac failure and strokes.

3. Dietary factors. Weight reduction should be encouraged, if appropriate, and advice regarding a lipid-lowering diet in those with unfavourable lipid profiles.

4. Physical activity. While it has proved difficult to study the effects of exercise in post-infarction patients, rehabilitation and exercise programmes, when tailored to the requirements of individual patients, should be encouraged.

Drug therapy

1. Antiplatelet therapy and anticoagulation. There have been a number of trials examining the benefits of aspirin and of oral anticoagulants post-MI. The majority have demonstrated lower reinfarction rates, reduced risk of subsequent cardiovascular death and reduced non-fatal MI. The majority of patients will receive aspirin following a MI although oral anticoagulants may be used in preference where other clinical indications co-exist, e.g. atrial fibrillation, left ventricular thrombus.

The optimal dose of aspirin has not been established beyond doubt, although 150 mg daily appears to afford benefit without significant adverse effects.

2. *Beta blockers.* A number of small and large-scale trials have demonstrated that beta blocker therapy reduces reinfarction rates and overall mortality post-MI. A meta-analysis of the results of 15 long-term trials demonstrated a 20% reduction in non-fatal reinfarction and a 20–25% reduction in overall mortality. Trials have included a variety of types of beta blocker including timolol, metoprolol and acebutalol, although there is no convincing evidence of additional benefit from any one single class of beta-blocking agents.

There is evidence that 'high risk' patients who have experienced electrical or mechanical complications secondary to MI have most to benefit from beta-blocking therapy. Beta blockers should be considered in all patients post-MI who do not have definite contraindications, e.g. asthma, advanced conduction disturbance, severe heart failure.

3. *Angiotensin-converting enzyme inhibitors.* There is convincing evidence that ACE inhibitors are of benefit in those patients with significant left ventricular dysfunction following MI. ACE inhibitors have been shown to limit left ventricular dilatation and dysfunction, thereby reducing morbidity and mortality.

A number of large-scale post-infarction trials have been conducted, including patients with symptomatic heart failure and those with asymptomatic left ventricular dysfuncion. The Acute Infarction Ramipril Efficacy (AIRE) study, for example, recruited 2006 patients with clinical signs or radiological evidence of heart failure. The results indicated that ACE inhibitor therapy with ramipril reduced overall mortality by 27%. The Survival and Ventricular Enlargement (SAVE) study, however, recruited patients on the basis of significant left ventricular systolic dysfunction (left ventricular ejection fraction 40% or less). There was a 19% reduction in overall mortality in the captopril-treated group, with evidence of a reduction in the incidence of recurrent MI.

ACE inhibitors should therefore be considered as secondary prevention in those patients who demonstrate clinical evidence of heart failure following MI and those where echocardiography demonstrates significant left ventricular dysfunction.

4. Calcium antagonists. There is little evidence to support the routine use of calcium antagonists post-infarction, although there is some evidence to support the use of agents such as verapamil or diltiazem in patients with small infarctions (e.g. non-Q-wave), who have contraindications to beta blockers.

5. Lipid-lowering therapy. The Scandanavian Simvastatin Survival Study (SSSS) demonstrated that simvastatin therapy in paients with total cholesterol levels between 5.5 and 8.0 mmol/l, and a history of prior MI or angina pectoris, reduced cardiovascular and all-cause mortality. The Cholesterol and Recurrent Events (CARE) study also confirmed the beneficial effects of statin therapy in post-infarction patients with rather lower cholesterol levels.

Statin drugs should be considered in post-infarction patients who have a total cholesterol level above 4.8 mmol/l or LDL-cholesterol above 3.2 mmol/l. There is emerging evidence that the beneficial effects of statin drugs may not only be as a result of cholesterol lowering, but that they may have a more direct role on cell proliferation, macrophage metabolism and immune function.

Further reading

Frishman WH. Secondary prevention with beta-adrenergic blockers and aspirin in ischeamic heart disease. *Current Opinion in Cardiology,* 1991; **6:** 567.

Pfeffer MA, Braunwald E, Moye LA *et al.* Effect of captopril on mortality and morbidity in patients with left ventricular dysfunction after MI. *New England Journal of Medicine,* 1992; **327:** 669.

The Acute Infarction Ramipril Efficacy (AIRE) Study Investigators. Effect of ramipril on mortality and morbidity of survivors of acute MI with clinical evidence of heart failure. *Lancet,* 1993; **342:** 821.

STROKE AND CARDIOVASCULAR DISEASE

Cardiac embolic strokes account for 1 out of every 5–6 ischaemic strokes. Out-patients presenting with ischaemic cerebral vascular events should be assessed for a potential cardiac source. In recent years, an increasing number of cardiac conditions have been identified as potential sources of cardiac embolism. Nevertheless part of the difficulty in determining the frequency of cardiac embolic stroke lies in the observation that there are significant limitations in making this clinical diagnosis. The following are potential cardiac sources of embolism:

Atrial fibrillation　　Atrial fibrillation is the most common cause of cardioembolic stroke, accounting for nearly half of the cases. Approximately 20% of these patients have rheumatic valve disease, 70% have non-valvular atrial fibrillation, and the remaining 10% have lone atrial fibrillation. Atrial fibrillation in association with valve disease carries an 18-fold increase in the risk of stroke, while non-valvular atrial fibrillation is estimated at approximately a 5-fold increase in risk. The role of anti-thrombolytic therapy and the management of atrial fibrillation has been discussed previously.

Rheumatic valve disease　　The relationship between mitral stenosis and thromboembolic complications is well recognized. Systemic thromboembolism occurs in 9–14% of patients with mitral stenosis with the majority of these events (up to 75%) being cerebral emboli. While systemic thromboembolic events related to mitral stenosis usually occur in association with atrial fibrillation, up to 20% occur in patients with sinus rhythm. Definite indications for anticoagulation include the presence of atrial fibrillation (chronic or paroxysmal) or a history of systemic thromboembolism (regardless of the patients rhythm). Other indications include the patient age of >40 years, and a dilated left atrium (>5.5 cm). A history of thromboembolism despite anticoagulation is a requirement of mitral valve surgery.

Myocardial infarction　　Stroke occurs as a complication in 2–4% of patients with MI, although the incidence of embolic stroke may be lower in the era of thrombotic therapy.

Thrombotic stroke is generally more common in anterior infarcts compared to inferior infarcts as most left ventricular thrombi occur over dyskinetic wall segments. Embolization is most common within the first 3–4 months with the highest risk during the first month. Anticoagulation can therefore be given prophylactically for all large, anterior infarcts for 3–6 months. After the initial 3–6 months post-infarction, a left ventricular aneurysm is considered chronic and stroke is an uncommon complication as mural thrombi are likely to be endothelized.

Dilated cardiomyopathy Patients with severely impaired left ventricular function and normal coronary arteries have a high incidence of intracardiac thrombus formation and embolic complications, on average 18% in patients not on anticoagulant therapy compared to no emboli in those on chronic anticoagulation therapy.

Prosthetic valves Systemic embolization occurs in both bioprosthetic and mechanical heart values at the rate of 1–4% a year. The risk for thromboembolism does not differ significantly between valve types. Nevertheless the absolute risk of thrombophlebitic events is higher for valves in the mitral position (2–3% a year) than in the aortic position (1–2% a year). Atrial fibrillation adds to this risk. Bioprostheses implanted in the mitral position should be anticoagulated for at least 3 months postoperatively even if the patient is in sinus rhythm. Nevertheless chronic anticoagulation is required if patients are in atrial fibrillation, if there is a left atrial thrombus present and there is a history of systemic embolic events. For both mechanical and bioprosthetic valves high-intensity anticoagulation does not necessarily further decrease the incidence of embolic complications.

Mitral valve prolapse This is a common cardiac condition, occurring in 4% of the general population. There is an association between mitral valve prolapse and cerebral ischaemic events in young adults, with a reported incidence of mitral valve prolapse of 30% of young patients with cerebral ischaemic events. The mechanism of stroke in such patients is not clearly understood, but it is felt that platelet–fibrin thrombi may form in the surface of redundant leaflet tissue which embolize. Anti-platelet therapy with aspirin is currently recommended for such patients.

Arteriosclerotic plaques in the aorta

The use of transoesophageal ECG has identified atherosclerotic 'debris' in the thoracic aorta. This refers to the appearance of increased echo density and thickening of the intima of the aorta, associated with irregularity or disruption of the intimal surface. There seems to be a strong association between atherosclerotic disease and ischaemic stroke.

Atrial septal aneurysm

An atrial septal aneurysm is redundancy of the tissue of the fossa ovalis that is at least 1.5 cm in length and demonstrates mobility, with maximal excursion between the left and right atrial of 1.5 cm. This condition occurs in 1% of the population, and diagnosis is frequently made by transoesophageal echocardiography.

Atrial septal aneurysms are associated with embolic events although the mechanism has not been defined clearly.

Patent foramen ovale

Patent foramen ovale is taken to be an anatomical variant, being found in 33% of persons by autopsy. In young patients with unexplained ischaemic stroke or transient ischaemic attacks, a patent foramen ovale can be found in 40–50%, compared to a 15% prevalence in controlled subjects. The finding of a patent foramen ovale, however, is insufficient evidence to presume a diagnosis of paradoxical embolism.

Spontaneous echo contrast

Spontaenous echo contrast refers to a smoke-like, swirling echo appearance seen within a cardiac chamber. It is generally thought to reflect stasis and is caused by the aggregation of red blood cells in a setting of low blood viscosity. It is commonly found in conditions such as atrial fibrillation, mitral stenosis, prosthetic mitral valves and severe left ventricular impairment. Spontaneous echo contrast has been associated with an increase in the incidence of thromboembolic complications. However, anticoagulation appears to have no correlation with the presence or absence of spontaneous echo contrast.

Bacterial endocarditis

The prevalence of ischaemic stroke in patients with infective endocarditis ranges between 15 and 20%, with most strokes occurring at presentation or within 48 hours of diagnosis. The appropriate treatment for stroke complicating endocarditis requires infection control and anticoagulation has no role in native valve endocarditis. Anticoagulation can in fact increase the risk of intracerebral haemorrhage in such cases.

Non-bacterial thrombotic endocarditis

This refers to valvular thrombi (usually <3 mm) associated with a pro-thrombotic state, for example malignancy or non-malignant wasting disease such as the acquired immunodeficiency syndrome. This is present in 0.5–1% of autopsies and is commonly found in patients with cancer. Heparin may be effective in preventing thromboembolic complications.

Mitral annular calcification

Calcification of the mitral annular ring refers to the chronic non-inflammatory, degenerative process involving the fibrous support structure of the mitral valve. The presence of mitral annular calcification is associated with a two-fold increase in the risk of stroke. Rather than a specific cause of stroke it may be a mark of a generalized arterial sclerosis or other cardiovascular disease.

Calcific aortic stenosis

Embolic complications are uncommon in patients with calcific aortic stenosis. Nevertheless emboli are small, occult or producing transient blindness. They are usually due to platelet or calcific emboli and have been associated with cardiac catheterization or percutaneous balloon valvuoplasty.

Cardiac tumours

Atrial myxoma is the most common primary cardiac tumour which can frequently embolize and cause stroke. The prevalence of atrial myxomas in patients with acute cerebrovascular events is approximately 1 in 750.

Intracardiac thrombus

Thrombus within the left ventricle occurs in a setting of acute MI, dilated cardiomyopathy and chronic left ventricular aneurysm. The majority of thrombi in the left atrium occur within the left atrial appendage and are commonly found in atrial fibrillation, mitral stenosis, prosthetic mitral valves, severe left ventricular dysfunction or left atrial dilatation.

Echocardiography is a powerful tool for the evaluation of cardioembolic stroke and transthoracic and transoesophageal echocardiography are complementary procedures. Transoesophageal echocardiography is particularly valuable in assessing mitral valve disease, left atrial thrombi, prosthetic valves and the detection of vegetations in suspected endocarditis.

Further reading

Lip GYH. Intracardiac thrombus formation in cardiac impairment: investigation and the role of anticoagulant therapy. *Postgraduate Medical Journal*, 1996; **72:** 731–8.

Lip GYH, Lowe GDO. Warfarin and aspirin as thromboprophylaxis in atrial fibrillation. *British Journal of Clinical Pharmacology*, 1996; **41:** 369–79.

Related topics of interest

Antithrombotic therapy in cardiovascular disorders (p. 13)
Cardiac tumours (p. 74)
Valve disease (p. 185)

SYNCOPE

Definition

Syncope is defined as a disturbance or loss of consciousness as a result of an abrupt reduction of blood flow to the brain, typically of short duration (seconds to minutes).

Causes   There are four main groups:

1. Obstruction to the circulation. Obstruction of emptying of the left heart (e.g. aortic stenosis, hypertrophic cardiomyopathy) or of the right heart (e.g. pulmonary stenosis, pulmonary hypertension or pulmonary embolism, Fallot's tetralogy) may cause syncope. Less commonly, the great vessels are obstructed, as in Takayasu's arteritis or subclavian steal; rarely impairment of venous filling occurs, e.g. cardiac tamponade. The cause of the problem is usually clinically apparent, except in left atrial myxoma or thrombus which may cause obstruction of the mitral orifice and diagnosis is usually then made by cardiac ultrasound.

2. Transient arrhythmias. Both tachyarrhythmia and bradyarrhythmia may cause syncope. Ventricular tachycardia commonly compromises cardiac output while supraventricular tachycardias may be better tolerated haemodynamically: if atrial fibrillation is documented in a patient with syncope then sick sinus syndrome (alternating tachycardia and bradycardia) or a pre-excitation syndrome, e.g. Wolff–Parkinson–White syndrome, should be considered.

Bradycardias, e.g. complete heart block or sinus node disease are important to identify since treatment using a pacemaker is usually very successful. Rarely, the carotid sinus becomes hypersensitive; stimulation by head movement may provoke bradycardia and syncope (carotid sinus syndrome). Dual chamber pacing is often effective; carotid sinus massage with ECG recording may aid bedside diagnosis. Syncopal attacks due to arrhythmias are usually abrupt in onset and offset and are associated with pallor during the attack and sometimes flushing on recovery (Stokes Adams attacks).

3. Vasovagal syndromes. Fainting is a common cause of syncope: both vagal slowing and reduced vasomotor tone (inappropriate vasodilatation) contribute to the haemodynamic disturbance. Attacks are usually associated with upright posture in stereotyped circumstances (e.g. with pain or the sight of blood, prolonged standing in a hot environment). The subject feels sweaty, nauseous and may yawn and often has a brief warning that fainting is imminent. Recovery is gradual over 5–10 minutes. Healthy people may have infrequent fainting attacks but if they occur frequently with little or no provocation the term malignant vasovagal syndrome is used. The diagnosis may be confirmed by provoking a typical syncopal attack during a tilt test, during which the patient is tilted to about 60 degrees on a tilt table, if confirmed, implantation of a dual chamber pacemaker may be helpful.

Patients with respiratory disease may have syncope after coughing, transient increases in intrathoracic pressure may stimulate the aortic baroreceptors leading to reflex bradycardia and vasodilatation (cough syncope). In elderly men, usually during nocturnal micturition, syncope may be provoked, raised intrathoracic and intra-abdominal pressure may reduce the venous return and emptying of the bladder may encourage reflex vasodilatation (micturition syncope).

4. Syncope associated with neurological disorders. A variety of neurological disorders may interfere with autonomic function, especially vagal control of heart rate and peripheral sympathetic vasoconstrictor fibres, e.g. paraplegia, diabetes mellitus, polyneuropathy. In some patients with tremor, bladder dysfunction and pupillary abnormalities, degeneration of the basal ganglia is associated with marked autonomic dysfunction (Shy–Drager syndrome or multi-system atrophy); idiopathic autonomic failure is also well recognized (Bradbury–Eggleton syndrome).

The distinguishing feature of these conditions is failure to maintain upright blood pressure with a fall in blood pressure on standing often most marked in the morning. Postural hypotension may also result from a number of drugs which interfere with autonomic function, e.g. phenothiazines and tricyclic antidepressants. In all these conditions reduction of plasma volume, e.g. due to diuretic therapy or following dehydration associated with intercurrent illness may markedly exacerbate symptoms.

Diagnosis

A detailed history is critical in reaching a diagnosis, eye witness accounts may be helpful. Distinction between syncope and epilepsy may be very difficult, disturbed brain function with stupor or confusion after the attack are typical of epilepsy. Laboured respiration with cyanosis and limb or facial movements during the attack are often helpful clues. In patients with transient cerebral ischaemic attacks the problem is usually identified as a result of short-lived focal neurological symptoms. When the hind brain circulation is disturbed typical symptoms are vertigo, dysarthria, diplopia and field defects. Confusingly cerebral anoxia during a syncopal attack may also provoke either focal or generalized epilepsy or transient focal neurological symptoms. Drop attacks may occur typically in elderly women: the patient describes suddenly finding herself on the pavement followed by an almost immediate recovery. Consciousness is not disturbed and the cause is a sudden loss of postural tone. The outlook is excellent. Hypoglycaemia is usually associated with sweating and recovery is typically more prolonged than with a syncopal attack.

Investigations

A resting ECG is essential, but a normal recording does not exclude an important rhythm disturbance which may be documented during a 24-hour

	(Holter) recording. In patients with infrequent symptoms a portable recorder, e.g. cardiomemo, may be necessary. Ultrasound examination of the heart and great vessels may help in assessment with patients with cardiac or arterial obstructive lesions.
Treatment	Treatment is usually directed at the cause. It is essential not to miss bradyarrhythmias since pacemaker implantation usually leads to a complete recovery.

Related topics of interest

Arrhythmias (p. 26–47)
Hypertension (p. 132)
Stroke and cardiovascular disease (p. 176)

VALVE DISEASE

Mitral stenosis

Aetiology. Rheumatic fever remains the most common cause of mitral stenosis, although the incidence is declining in the Western world.

Acute rheumatic valvulitis results in inflammatory changes which in the long-term lead to scarring, thickening, shortening and deformity of the mitral valve cusps and the chordae. Inflammation along the margins of the leaflets leads to fusion of the commisures.

The causes of mitral stenosis include:

- Rheumatic fever.
- Congenital (associated ASD-Lutembacher's syndrome).
- Mucopolysaccharoidoses (e.g. Hurler's syndrome).
- Prosthetic valve.
- Malignant carcinoid.

Mitral stenosis causes a diastolic pressure gradient between the left atrium and ventricle, and therefore elevation in left atrial pressure and left atrial dilatation. In turn this causes pulmonary venous, pulmonary arterial and right heart hypertension, with pulmonary oedema.

Symptoms. The patient may be asymptomatic although symptoms may included dyspnoea, fatigue, palpitations, haemoptysis, cough, dysphagia, hoarseness (Ortner's syndrome) and angina. Dyspnoea is the most frequent symptom, but haemoptysis, ankle oedema, and embolic events are also frequent.

Signs. Malar flush, small volume pulse, atrial fibrillation, parasternal heave (right ventricular hypertrophy and dilatation) and tapping apex beat. Auscultation may reveal an opening snap, loud first heart sound (soft or absent if cusps are calcified and immobile) and a mid-diastolic murmur with presystolic accentuation (absent in atrial fibrillation).

Longstanding and severe mitral valve disease may lead to pulmonary hypertension with a high pitched pulmonary diastolic murmur (Graham Steel murmur).

Investigations

- ECG. Atrial fibrillation or evidence of left atrial enlargement may be present.
- CXR. Left atrial enlargement is suggested by a prominent left atrial appendage, straight left heart border, double left atrial shadow and carinal angle > 100°. Calcification of the mitral valve may be visible.
- ECHO. Left atrium is enlarged and hardening or calcification of mitral leaflets seen. Doppler measurements are used to estimate the mitral valve gradient and area. Mitral valve area below 1 cm^2 suggests severe mitral stenosis. Transoesophageal echocardiography provides more detailed assessment of the mitral valve.
- Cardiac catheter. Simultaneous tracings of the pulmonary artery wedge pressure and left ventricular pressure allow assessment of the mitral valve gradient. Cardiac catheterization is rarely needed to establish a diagnosis, but is performed in older patients requiring surgical management or before balloon valvuloplasty.

Management. Atrial fibrillation in the context of mitral stenosis is associated with a high incidence of thromboembolism and these patients should be anticoagulated. Digoxin, diuretics and vasodilators e.g. nitrates may improve the symptoms. If pulmonary hypertension develops or pulmonary congestion persists then intervention is required. Balloon valvuloplasty is the proceedure of choice, although open surgical valvotomy or valve replacement may still be required.

Mitral balloon valvuloplasty should be avoided where there is significant mitral regurgitation or where the mitral valve is heavily calcified.

Mitral regurgitation

Mitral regurgitation may be secondary to abnormalities of the mitral valve annulus, leaflets, the chordae or the papillary muscles. Common causes include:
- Functional (dilated left ventricle).

- Rheumatic fever.
- Infectious endocarditis.
- Mitral calcification.
- Mitral valve prolapse.
- Chordal rupture.
- Papillary muscle rupture (acute).

Any condition causing left ventricular dilatation can lead to mitral regurgitation. Primary disease of the mitral valve also causes regurgitation. Ischaemia, hypertension, cardiomyopathies, rheumatic fever, connective tissue disease, collagen disease, valvular prolapse and valvular degeneration are the commonest precipitants.

Symptoms. Patients may be asymptomatic for many years although acute mitral regurgitation e.g. papillary muscle rupture often leads to a rapid clinical deterioration. Dyspnoea is normally the predominant symptom.

Signs. Atrial fibrillation may be present with a displaced heaving apex and a pan-systolic murmur at the apex which radiates to the axilla. There may be a systolic thrill and third heart sound. The first heart sound is quiet in severe mitral regurgitation.

Investigations.

- ECG. Left atrial enlargement and in 50% of cases left ventricular hypertrophy.
- CXR. Cardiomegaly, left atrial enlargement and signs of pulmonary venous congestion.
- ECHO. Assessment of left atrial size, left ventricular size and function and evidence of leaflet prolapse. Doppler will establish site and size of regurgitation jet.
- Cardiac catheter. Left ventricular angiography will demonstrate the severity of the regurgitation and right heart catheterization allows assessment of the pulmonary artery wedge pressure. The size of the 'v' wave depends on the severity of the mitral regurgitation and left atrial size.

Management. Medical treatment with diuretics, digoxin, ACE inhibitors and vasodilators is normally effective in controlling symptoms. Patients with atrial fibrillation should be anticoagulated, unless there is a contraindication.

Mitral valve repair or replacement should be considered in severe mitral regurgitation or where symptoms persist despite medical therapy.

Aortic stenosis

Aetiology

- Degenerative calcific aortic stenosis.
- Rheumatic heart disease.
- Congenital (bicuspid aortic valve).
- Atherosclerosis (severe hyperlipidaemia).

Aortic stenosis commonly co-exists with aortic regurgitation.

Pathophysiologically aortic stenosis produces a systolic pressure gradient between the left ventricle and aorta, and subsequent left ventricular hypertrophy. The end stage of this process is left ventricular failure and death.

Symptoms. Patients are often asymptomatic until the aortic stenosis is severe. Symptoms include dyspnoea, angina and exertional syncope. Systemic emboli may also lead to retinal or cerebral symptoms.

Signs. Clinical findings include slow rising pulse, a thrusting apex beat, an ejection systolic murmur at the left sternal edge radiating into the carotids, a fourth heart sound and reduced aortic closure sound. The second sound is inaudible when the valve is calcified. There may be a left ventricular heave and palpable systolic thrill.

Investigations

- ECG. Left axis deviation and LVH or LBBB.
- CXR. Left ventricular enlargement, aortic valve calcification and post stenotic dilatation of the ascending aorta.
- ECHO. Bicuspid aortic valve, left ventricular hypertrophy, aortic calcification. Doppler studies assess aortic velocity to allow estimation of the aortic valve gradient.
- Cardiac catheter. Assessment of left ventricular function, the withdrawal gradient across the

aortic valve and the diagnosis of coronary artery disease.

Management. Antibiotic prophylaxis is mandatory for dental and other surgical procedures. Aortic valve replacement is considered when the aortic stenosis is severe (greater than 60 mm Hg) or when the gradient is smaller but the patient is symptomatic.

Aortic regurgitation

The most common causes of aortic regurgitation are rheumatic fever and infectious endocarditis, although there are numerous causes and associations.

Acute

- Acute rheumatic fever.
- Infectious endocarditis.
- Aortic dissection.
- Ruptured aneurysm of the Sinus of Valsalva.

Chronic

- Rheumatic fever.
- Bicuspid aortic valve.
- Infectious endocarditis.
- Severe hypertension.
- Syphilis.
- Marfan's Syndrome.
- Ankylosing spondylitis.
- Rheumatoid arthritis.

Pathophysiologically, aortic regurgitation volume loads the left ventricle leading to compensatory dilatation and hypertrophy. In latter stages left ventricular failure occurs. Acute aortic regurgitation causes frank pulmonary oedema and cardiogenic shock. Chronic aortic regurgitation is often asymptomatic for many years, but can present with cardiac failure or angina.

Symptoms. Patients are frequently asymptomatic, although dyspnoea and angina are common when the aortic regurgitation is severe.

Signs. The pulse is collapsing and there is a wide pulse pressure.The apex is displaced and thrusting. Auscultation reveals an immediate high pitched diastolic murmur heard loudest at the lower left sternal edge in expiration. Pistol-shot femorals are associated with severe incompetence. The following eponymous signs may also be present;

- Quincke's. Capillary pulsation in the nail beds.
- Corrigan's. Visible arterial pulsation in the neck.
- De Musset's. Head nodding related to the heart beat.
- Durozier's. Systolic bruit over the femoral arteries.

Investigations
- ECG. LVH (volume overload).
- CXR. Left ventricular enlargement and possibly dilatation of the ascending aorta.
- ECHO. Left ventricle and aortic root may be dilated. Diastolic fluttering of the mitral valve leaflets may be seen in severe aortic regurgitation. Colour flow and continuous wave Doppler studies will allow assessment of the severity of the aortic regurgitation.
- Cardiac catheter. Aortic root injection demonstrates reflux of contrast into the left ventricle. Cardiac catheter studies are usually unnecessary to make the diagnosis, but are performed preoperatively to assess left ventricular function and delineate coronary anatomy and aortic dilatation.

Management. The underlying cause should be treated if possible e.g. infectious endocarditis. Symptoms normally occur when the left ventricular function deteriorates, although aortic valve replacement at this stage does not normally restore the function and is associated with higher morbidity and mortality. Valve replacement should be considered before significant deterioration in the left ventricular function, as indicated by haemodynamic and echocardiographic assessment. Aortic valve replacement is required once symptoms occur or if progressive asymptomatic left ventricular dilatation is identified.

Tricuspid stenosis

This is an uncommon lesion and is usually secondary to rheumatic heart disease. Tricuspid stenosis is rarely an isolated lesion and is mostly associated with mitral and aortic lesions. It is occasionally seen in the carcinoid syndrome.

Signs and symptoms. If sinus rhythm is maintained a prominent jugular venous 'a' wave is seen, although atrial fibrillation is commonly present. There is a rumbling diastolic murmur at the left sternal edge which is louder on inspiration. An opening snap may be present. There may be hepatomegaly, ascites and peripheral oedema.

Investigations

- ECG. Right atrial enlargement.
- CXR. Prominent right atrial bulge.
- ECHO. Tricuspid valve is thickened and immobile.
- Cardiac catheter. Diastolic pressure gradient between the right atrium and right ventricle.

Management. Medical therapy with diuretics may be effective, although tricuspid valvotomy and valve replacement are often necessary.

Tricuspid regurgitation

Functional tricuspid regurgitation may occur as a result of right ventricular dilatation which occurs in pulmonary hypertension. Primary tricuspid regurgitation may result from rheumatic heart disease, carcinoid syndrome, Ebstein's anomaly and atrioventricular cushion defects. It may also result from endocarditis of the tricuspid valve, a condition which is associated with intravenous drug abuse.

Signs and symptoms. The patient may describe symptoms of right heart failure. Atrial fibrillation is common and a large jugular venous 'cv' wave is seen with a palpable and pulsatile liver. The right ventricular impulse may be palpable and a pan-systolic murmur is audible at the left sternal edge which is loudest on inspiration.

Mitral valve prolapse is often associated with atypical chest pains and palpitations.

Examination reveals a mid-systolic click and a mid-late systolic murmur.

Management. Functional regurgitation is usually managed with medical therapy although organic regurgitation occasionally requires annuloplasty, repair or valve replacement.

Pulmonary stenosis

This is normally a congenital lesion and may be associated with a VSD (Fallot's Tetralogy) or as part of the Rubella syndrome (congenital heart disease, mental retardation and blindness). Pulmonary stenosis may be valvar, supravalvar or subvalvar.

Signs and symptoms. Severe pulmonary stenosis may result in syncope, dyspnoea and symptoms of right heart failure. Mild stenosis may be asymptomatic.

A right ventricular heave may be present with a harsh pulmonary mid-systolic murmur which is loudest in inspiration. There may be a thrill and the pulmonary closure sound is usually delayed and soft.

Investigations

- ECG. Normal or evidence of right atrial and ventricular hypertrophy.
- CXR. Prominent pulmonary artery due to post-stenotic dilatation.
- Cardiac catheter. Systolic pressure gradient across the stenosis.

Management. Pulmonary balloon dilatation or open valvotomy may be required.

Pulmonary regurgitation

This normally results from dilatation of the pulmonary valve ring secondary to pulmonary hypertension. A decrescendo diastolic murmur is heard, the Graham Steel murmur, which may be indistinguishable from aortic regurgitation. The patient is rarely symptomatic and treatment is rarely indicated.

Related topic of interest

Cardiac failure (p. 48)

VENOUS AND PULMONARY THROMBOEMBOLISM

The incidence rate of deep venous thrombosis (DVT) in the general population is between 48 and 162 per 100 000 population and the rate of pulmonary embolism (PE) is 25–51 per 1 000 000 per year. PE is the cause of death or a major contributing factor in 3–16% of patients who die in hospital. However, in less than one-third of cases was the diagnosis suspected before death.

Risk factors for venous thromboembolism

These can be summarized into the following broad categories.

1. Clinical factors. This includes previous venous thromboembolism, poor mobility (bed rest, stroke, paralysis, trauma, surgery), malignancy, varicose veins, increased age, heart failure, oestrogen use, central venous catheters, pregnancy or the puerperium, inflammatory bowel disease, etc.

Patient groups at risk of DVT and deep PE without prophylaxis include the following: Hip fracture or surgery (40–60%), stroke (20–50%), major trauma (40–80%), spinal cord injury (60–80%), gynaecological surgery (20–40% malignant, 5–10% benign), myocardial infarction (15–40%), intensive care unit (30%), general abdominal surgery (20–40%).

2. Coagulation system factors. Myeloproliferative disorders (e.g. polycythemia, primary thrombocytosis), abnormal factor V (resulting in resistance to activated protein C), antiphospholipid antibody syndrome, deficiencies of antithrombin III, protein C, protein S, etc. are all risk factors. More rare causes are homocysteinaemia, heparin-induced thrombocytopenia with thrombosis and dysfibrinogenaemia.

A large proportion of hospitalized medical and surgical admissions are therefore at increased risk of thromboembolic complications. Nevertheless, this condition is largely preventable. The most efficient way is the routine use of thromboprophylaxis in high- and moderate-risk patients. DVT prophylaxis has been demonstrated to reduce the incidence of venous thromboembolism by as much as 70% with significant reduction in morbidity and all cause mortality.

Prevention of DVT and PE

Oral anticoagulants have been shown to be effective in preventing DVT and PE mortality. These have been given in many different regimes, including a mini-dose warfarin regimes, fixed dose regimes, standard anticoagulation, etc. The rationale for mini-dose or fixed regimes would be the avoidance of regular International Normalized Ratio (INR) monitoring.

The most common prophylactic treatment regimen is with subcutaneous heparin as prophylaxis, e.g. 5000 IU b.d. or t.i.d. Routine use of oral anticoagulants as prophylaxis is most common in high risk patients including those undergoing hip or knee surgery, surgery for hip fracture and in trauma patients with spinal cord injury or leg fracture.

Other measures such as compression (TED) stockings, passive calf muscle exercises and continued ambulation/early mobilization are useful.

Treatment of DVT and PE

The objectives of treatment are the cessation of thrombus extension, prevention of symptomatic PE and the reduction in chest or leg symptoms associated with initial events. It is also intended that treatment results in the prevention of recurrence after the initial thrombotic process has been suppressed. There should also be a reduction in the risk of post-phlebitic complications and prevention of thromboembolic pulmonary hypertension.

The usual treatment of DVT or PE is an initial course of intravenous heparin, or full-dose subcutaneous heparin, for 5–10 days, followed by oral anticoagulants for at least 3 months. The necessity of initial heparinization is to allow immediate anticoagulation, as warfarin takes 2–3 days to achieve inhibition of vitamin-K dependant coagulation factors and achieve systemic anticoagulant effect. The target INR for treating DVT or PE is between 2.0 and 3.0.

Further reading

Kearon C, Hirsh J. Management of anticoagulation before and after elective surgery. *New England Journal of Medicine,* 1997; **336:** 1506–11.

Related topic of interest

Antithrombotic therapy in cardiovascular disorders (p. 13)

INDEX